The Handbook
of Natural Beauty

The Handbook
of Natural Beauty

By *Virginia Castleton*

Rodale Press, Inc., Emmaus, Pa. 18049

Printed in the United States of America on recycled paper

Library of Congress Cataloging in Publication Data

Castleton, Virginia.
    The handbook of natural beauty.

    Includes index.
    1. Beauty, Personal. 2. Cosmetics. I. Title.
RA778.C243   646.7'02'4042   75-25828
ISBN 0-87857-100-0 (Hardcover)
ISBN 0-87857-217-1 (Paperback)

  14 16 18 20 19 17 15 13   hardcover
         6 8 10 9 7   paperback

Dedication

To Sybil—with memories aplenty of a shared childhood that never got lost.

Acknowledgments

Writing this book has been a memorable experience because of the close cooperation I have enjoyed from the staff of Rodale Press.

I especially want to thank Charles Gerras for his inspiring guidance and Anne Moyer for her dedicated assistance.

My gratitude also to Mark Bricklin, Executive Editor of *Prevention,* who initiated this project.

But to all at Rodale Press goes my deeply felt gratitude for the keen and abiding interest in this book.

Other Books
 by Virginia Castleton

Look Younger, Look Prettier
My Secrets of Natural Beauty
The Calendar Book of Natural Beauty

Contents

Introduction

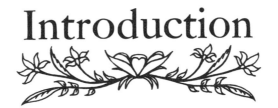

Every woman needs a beauty manual to consult for self-help in smoothing roughened skin, removing dark circles from under her eyes and for a multitude of other cosmetic problems that arise daily. She needs a reliable source for quick, effective advice when her lips suddenly crack after trying a new lipstick, or her hair begins to thin and becomes lifeless and brittle. As any woman will tell you, these disturbances are a frustrating part of everyday living. So the solution must be sensible and right at hand.

As beauty editor of *Prevention* magazine, the largest health publication in the world, and from continually delving into the whys and wherefores of skin conditions, overweight problems and other disturbances, I have accumulated in my files a wealth of material that should be available to any woman who cares about her appearance and who wants more satisfaction out of her days; any woman who always wants to look and feel her very best.

The beauty-conscious woman develops the know-how to deal with any and all of the cosmetic problems that assault her. Free from all worries about her appearance, she can concentrate on other matters.

I believe a book like this one is long overdue, for it is a

handbook of information to which you can turn when the appearance of any area of your body bewilders, annoys, or distracts you. While it is true that magazines and newspapers today carry an impressive amount of information on care of the body, diet, and beauty tips, this day to day means of supplying information is not really satisfactory for long time referral.

During April you may see an article on dry skin care in a periodical. But your skin may be behaving nicely that month, and in June or July begin to resemble a flaky strudel. If you haven't kept the article, or cannot remember where you put it, you are without the means of helping yourself to overcome your problem.

There are also beauty books available that teach you to become a kitchen cosmetologist. But the ones I have seen include undesirable products. By eliminating objectionable items like glycerin, alkaline soaps, borax, mineral oil and other petroleum products, I have kept the concoctions in this book on the level of simple put-togethers and totally uncomplicated formulas. You needn't become a chemist in using these means to enhance yourself, and you *will* look and feel better.

In this manual you will find the answers you seek when you look into the mirror and see premature wrinkling, early graying of the hair, or a surly blemish of unknown origin. Sections are presented in the order of the most frequently occurring problems.

The solutions to your distresses are not shrouded in vague terms in this book. Here, in non-technical language, is information based on years of medical and nutritional research and personal interviews with women who have helped themselves out of a variety of body faults by searching tirelessly until they found an answer.

Defensive beauty practices are necessary for most of us.

That is, we must work to prevent various cosmetic problems that tend to develop due to poor nutrition, pollutants in the air that can fill delicate pore openings, and other assaults made upon our bodies by the hectic pace of modern living.

Unless she takes time to care for her hair and complexion, and unless she gives some thought to keeping her body young and active, a woman can arrive at 30 looking 40. The aging process in itself is an illness, according to biologists, but one that can be postponed or delayed, by proper attention to the body. The drama of reversing the aging syndrome is a stimulating experience. When you improve your appearance, you also boost your morale. And we all function better and are more comfortable when we know we have presented our best to our critical selves and to the world.

Read through this book with the realization that, while every person is distinctively different from everyone else, there are areas of similarity and problems of common origin that can affect us all in varying degrees. And next to the problem is the solution that has helped so many women in their search for greater beauty, health, and comfort. Here, then, is your own guide to beauty.

Chapter 1

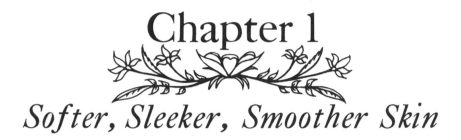

Softer, Sleeker, Smoother Skin

Skin is the efficient body covering that protects our inner parts and guards their processes, gauges our temperature needs and reflects internal disorders. It is easy to care for and responsive to good treatment. And it influences our lives socially, sexually and healthfully.

The four layers of the skin are constantly growing and renewing themselves. The epidermis, or outer layer, should be flexible and elastic to accommodate the needs of your body. It is this layer that constantly flakes off, being replaced by cells from the layers underneath. Not to realize this is inviting problems. We need a small amount of friction occasionally to remove the dead, flaked-off cells. If this layer of debris is not removed in time, there is trouble in the form of enlarged, clogged pores and lifeless looking skin that cannot breathe.

Actually, removing this layer of skin is a most rewarding activity. It always brings a pleasurable glow of feeling immaculate, as well as acquiring an instantly improved appearance. There is no discomfort involved.

There are many methods and many preparations that have been created to do this job. Which you choose doesn't matter as long as you find an effective way to keep your skin breathing, to keep the lifeline open from the deepest underlying layers to the one everybody sees.

What's Your Skin Type?

To bring out your skin's best qualities, you must first know its type.

Generally we recognize three skin types: oily, dry and normal. Within that range great variety can exist. In fact, combinations of the three can and often do occur; sometimes different areas of one person's face harbor two, or all three conditions.

To test individually for the different types and to determine, first, if you have a dry or oily skin, wash your face upon arising, rinse with warm and then cool water and blot dry. Leave the skin free of makeup for at least an hour. Then press a clean tissue against the entire facial surface. Don't rub; merely press firmly to determine if there will be surface oils the tissue will absorb. Now examine the tissue. Your skin's degree of oiliness can be determined by the amount of grease on the tissue. The total absence of oil will indicate a dry skin. (You may have already determined that your skin is dry because of its unnatural tautness after washing it.) Some may confuse normal and slightly dry skins, but the former can benefit from external dry skin treatment, so don't be afraid to lavish care on it.

Normal skin may or may not have a slight bit of oil on it an hour after washing it. It will be a comfortable skin, with no unpleasant pulling sensation.

The pH factor is something that one hears and reads more and more about in relation to the body. PH refers to the body's acid-alkaline balance. The healthy skin has an acid mantle that protects it from bacterial invasion.

The mantle can have a pH range anywhere from 5.2 to 6 within a scale of 4.5 to 7.5 on Squibbs' nitrazine paper, a good testing device. The lower number represents the acid side of the scale, and the higher denotes an alkaline state.

Cosmetics

Throughout history women have coated themselves with everything from mud and grease to guard against insects, to delicate pomades for softening and scenting the skin. Complicated formulas have been devised to keep the skin youthful—some have succeeded and some have been fatal. The lucky women used flower lotions, simple unguents, fruits, vegetables and herbs. Those who used heavy metals like lead and arsenic in their concoctions often ended up as casualties.

One of the most attractive women I've met, an actress with the *Comedie Francaise,* kept her skin supple and gleaming with a thin mixture of olive oil and lemon juice, and with no other makeup whatsoever offstage.

Your skin is a barometer of health. Reflected here will be indications of what is happening within your body. According to your diet, sleeping habits, and the kind of life you lead, this organ of expression can be gleaming with health and beauty or dull and suggestive of *malaise.*

Some of the most expensive commercial cosmetics contain harmful ingredients, yet they are popular. Why the great demand for these destructive products? Cigarettes are cited by the Surgeon General's office as harmful to your health, yet they are on the market to be sold to an informed but indifferent public. Alcohol is known to cause liver damage, and still it is consumed by Americans everywhere. The answer, of course, is that these items bring in millions of dollars to the manufacturers. Through the miracle of mass media, products are glamorized and made irresistible to an unwary public. If a product gives us the results that advertisers make us believe we want, we shrug off warnings that the product may be unsafe. Thus, with the image of the ideal woman ever before her, modern woman strives for physical perfection by trying every new cosmetic on the market. And though illnesses and injuries have resulted from the use of some cosmetics, there has been no major epidemic, and the injuries that do occur as a result of damaging ingredients in some cosmetics are barely publicized.

At the same time, we don't say that *all* commercial cosmetics are damaging. Some are very helpful in concealing conditions that cannot be helped otherwise—and as long as there is no damage to the body, these cosmetics seem acceptable. Unfortunately, most of us require more than just "getting by." The majority of people using cosmetics are searching for a real and lasting answer to an actual physical problem—and no inert, non-nutritious substance is going to satisfy that need. Fortunately, for those people who do not have the time or inclination to prepare their own cosmetics, or at least a portion of them, there is a variety of natural cosmetics coming onto the market.

For the first time in years I have been able to use a lipstick without having my lips peel, bleed and flake. And the California based company which produces it has my blessings. It is sold only in health food shops, and to my way of thinking, it *is* healthy. I tried just about every brand on the market before finding this one, called *Cosmetic Naturals,* by Gwen.

Hypoallergenic Cosmetics

Every shop selling hypoallergenic products should have a chart available listing the ingredients in the products.

This is not to say that a list of ingredients automatically insures safety to a person sensitive to cosmetics. But at least you will have an idea of what you are putting on your skin. Hypoallergenic products are supposedly free of irritants and allergens, but they still contain numerous chemicals.

I was, frankly, appalled when I consulted the chart for a popular hypoallergenic product recently and learned what was in it. The following are just a few of the ingredients in hypoallergenic cosmetics of all types from night creams to eyeliners: sodium borate, glyceryl monostearate, methyl and propyl parahydroxybenzoate, mineral oil, polyoxyethylene sorbitan mon-oleate, and homolog menthyl salicylate. These items are just a part of the chemical feast you are applying to your skin whether you use hypoallergenic cosmetics or the usual commercial types.

I cannot explain why some people are allergic to some brands of cosmetics and not to others, any more than I can tell you why some people are allergic to strawberries and others are not. Remember, each person is different from all others, and some people's systems simply cannot tolerate certain compounds, which others can. One ingredient more than any other that has proved sensitizing in cosmetics is perfume, which isn't needed in the first place in creams that are rubbed into the body. Not only can perfume irritate and cause an allergic reaction, but when the perfumed skin is exposed to the sun, it might darken or splotch.

Natural Cosmetics

Health food shops, as wonderful as they can be, are still commercial enterprises. Most of them genuinely try to provide health and beauty products that are superior to those sold in supermarkets, drug stores, and department stores. But like other retailers, they have to accept the word of the manufacturer on the safety and merit of products. Even if the product is properly labeled, an individual may still have an allergic reaction to a specific ingredient permitted by law in a preparation.

Fissured skin, for example, could come from the inclusion of glycerin in a cosmetic preparation. Glycerin is abundantly used in cosmetics today, even though it can irritate and dry the skin. It is a by-product of soap manufacture and, according to Charles Perry, English nutritionist and beautician, is toxic in cumulative amounts.

Glycerin mixed with water or some other suitable liquid acts as a moisturizing agent when it is applied to the skin. But rather than act as a humectant, which attracts moisture from the air, glycerin first draws whatever moisture it can from the underlying tissues of the skin itself. Because it absorbs this water from the tissues, glycerin keeps the body in a state of dependence. As long as glycerin is applied, the external skin surface will have some semblance of elasticity and softness. But when the applications cease, the skin takes on a dry, raspy feel. Any preparation containing glycerin, then, can be damaging to delicate skin tissues. Though our grandmothers had many delightful, marvelously effective beauty aids, they also had a few, such as glycerin water, that could be damaging.

Homemade Cosmetics

One of the main reasons for preparing your own creams, lotions and other beauty treatments is to have fresh, unpreserved ingredients. But when you use fresh foods for your cosmetics you must realize that cosmetics made from these items are just as perishable as though they had been prepared for a meal.

Remember that natural cosmetics prepared in your own

kitchen come from foods that supply nutrients, not preservatives. They should, therefore, be treated as foods and
not be expected to stay fresh any longer than an unrefriger-
ated food. A fresh strawberry and cream facial is lovely,
and does wonderful things for a muddy complexion. But
if you leave this mixture at room temperature for 24 hours,
you'll have sour milk and fermented berries.

Oils, vinegars and lanolin mixtures will keep longer.
But where kitchen cosmetics are concerned, treat them as
you would any food. Make up only the amount you will
use right away and realize that preservatives do nothing
for your body.

General Care

Perhaps you are one of those lucky souls blessed with a
naturally beautiful complexion. If so, even your fine skin
needs general maintenance to keep it soft and fresh.

This section is devoted to delightful concoctions you can
whip up to help maintain a glowing, radiant complexion.

General Care/Strawberries

The use of strawberries in beauty preparations is a practice of long standing, and their aid to the complexion has
been firmly established. Ancient beauty recipes speak of
crushing berries and oatmeal, berries and cream, and other
combinations to produce varying effects.

Since their pH is the same as that of our skin, they have
become one of my weaknesses. Other women may succumb
to a new makeup or lipstick, but I really have a weakness
for these incredible berries—not so much to eat as to wear.
My skin really sparkles after a strawberry facial.

I've been so turned on by the value of a strawberry facial

that I've surrendered to their lure in far-away places—*especially* in far away places where I know they have been organically grown. In a marketplace in Helsinki, Finland, I bought a box of strawberries grown in the volcanic ash of nearby mountains. Standing in the square I ate the incredibly sweet berries (yes, they were first rinsed with a bottle of clear, spring water) and absentmindedly rubbed one into my skin. It was a chilly, late summer day and everyone was bundled up with babushkas and wraps so I didn't think I'd be too conspicuous.

We moved on to the area in the square where Russia's first cosmonaut, Gagarin, was addressing a youth group. People began edging away from me and eventually I realized they believed I had some dread disease, like measles, due to my strawberry facial. I found another bottle of water, rinsed my face and got back in time to hear the promise of pie in the sky from the cosmonaut to a rather hostile audience. But I did profit from my strawberry facial, and I've never forgotten the incredible sweetness of the berries, even though my own home state of Louisiana is known for the old fashioned delectable strawberry that remains small, firm, and only faintly red, but totally delicious.

A really old practice was to mash a cup of the juicy sun-ripened berries in an equal amount of water. This was applied, before retiring, to the face, arms, shoulders, bosom and hands.

The softening and cleansing effect of this recipe is supposed to take place while you sleep, and the dried mixture is washed away in the morning. According to the original recipe, "After rinsing away the dried strawberry juice, your shoulders and bosom will be as fair as any maiden's." That's a big promise, but if you will settle for less dramatic benefits, you will still be ahead.

Fresh Strawberry Mask

The strawberry mask is very effective for softening and lightening skin that has grown yellow-tinged, or has taken too deep a tan, but it requires patience and repeated applications to do its work most effectively. Wash and hull a handful of fresh, sun-ripened strawberries. Mash them with a wooden spoon into a glass custard cup. Now, gather the liquefied fruit and pat the mixture onto the face and neck area. Allow this to dry before rinsing away with warm water.

For those with a sensitive skin, mash the strawberries and beat in an equal amount of water before applying to the skin.

One of my yoga teachers sailed into her fiftieth year with limbs and body as flexible, as slender and as well moulded as they had been 20 years earlier. True, she spent hours out of each day performing yoga movements as she taught her numerous classes, but her body was as youthful as those of many of the women she taught, who were half her age.

Her complexion was equally outstanding, for this woman was eager to learn and practice all of the benefits that come from natural living. With only a small backyard at her home, and that in shade, she devised a method of growing strawberries in a huge urn that had pocket-like openings all over it, and placed the huge pot on her porch. She set strawberry plants into all the slots and reaped an ample harvest of the juicy, skin-tingling berries.

This woman considered a strawberry and cream application, used frequently, a beauty aid worth the effort of growing strawberries in such a restricted manner. Seeing her smooth face, who would question her approach to skin preservation?

If your internal nutrition is sensible, your composure serene, and you top these attributes with a strawberry-

and-cream facial mask, you, too, may well avoid early wrinkling, and even postpone the tendency to wrinkle at any age.

Strawberry-and-Cream Facial Mask

Select fresh, well ripened whole strawberries, just in from the berry patch. Wash and hull carefully. Shake the strawberries dry and mash several of them in a glass custard cup. Mix in an equal amount of fresh, rich cream and pat this onto the face with tapping movements. Apply the mixture to all parts of the face, and if you don't mind the bother, cover the throat and neck for additional benefits.

Be ready to rest for 30 minutes while this mask remains in place and does its work. This is truly a luxurious facial mask, and the combination of rest and skin nutrition does wonders for a tired skin. Save this one for special days when you won't be rushed or disturbed, and when you can fully enjoy the rest period.

Would you have guessed that you can get a peaches and cream complexion from peaches and cream? It's a fact. Just blend some ripe peach with a dab of golden cream. Massaged into a nondescript complexion, it will tinge the cheeks with a blushing glow.

General Care/Attar of Roses

Heavy creams and lotions can be stultifying to delicate skin tissues. There are times when we all feel the need to apply a blanket of nutrition to the skin in the hope of instant renewal, or to atone for past neglect. But it is the day to day care that will bring rewards. Like using a delicately scented water that refreshes and lifts the spirit because it makes one *feel* lovely.

One of the most beautifully scented and cherished flower

waters of all time has its basis in attar of roses. This is a difficult scent to prepare unless you have a large quantity of unsprayed roses. The costly oil from which the water can be made generally sells for a prohibitively high one hundred and twenty-five dollars an ounce. If you've enough roses whose petals would fill a small basket, then this could be a do-it-yourself project of great reward.

So, if you have the patience and a sense of adventure, plus a rose garden, you can produce your own attar of roses and feel like a sultan's daughter in the sheer beauty you can create by using the attar in a lighter rose water mixture. The discovery of rose oil was made by a Persian princess whose father, the Grand Mogul, had filled his canals with roses. The princess noticed the strange film floating on the water surface, and because it was so fragrant, ordered it to be collected and the oil squeezed out. The production of rose *otto,* or attar of roses, at Shiraz dates from this event in the seventeenth century.

Attar of Roses

To prepare your own attar of roses, pick all the roses you can and carefully remove the petals. Remove any foreign substance from the petals and drop them into a large earthenware jar or pot. Cover the petals with distilled water and then place a fine screen over the top of the vessel, to prevent insects from getting in. Set the pot in the sunshine every day and bring it indoors at night. Eventually the essential oil from the rose petals will appear on the surface of the water.

Use cotton swabs to lift the matter off the water. Squeeze the oil from the cotton tips into a small glass vial with a stopper or lid. Continue the process each day thereafter until no more oil arises. Then use this precious oil as a basis for the following rose water.

Rose Water

Dissolve one teaspoon of rose oil in one pint of ethyl alcohol, which has been warmed by placing the container in hot water. Pour the combined oil and alcohol into a two-gallon container, and add one and three-fourths gallons of distilled water that has been heated to just below the boiling point. Cork the container and shake gently and then thoroughly until the mixture becomes cold.

Now you have a winter's supply of scented body lotion to use after a bath, or just as a refreshing sponge solution. You will want to bottle the rose water in smaller containers that are more convenient to handle. Because there is no fixative agent in this, you might want to share your rose water with friends, so it can be used before it begins to lose its scent.

General Care/Milk of Roses

Sometimes a helpful cosmetic item is discovered that proves to be so effective and practical that it becomes legendary. In an earlier century, one such product was called a complexion paste. Obviously, advertising was an unpracticed art in those days, for paste is about the last thing today's market could sell as a beauty aid.

But the lovely and useful concoction I have in mind is full of so many beneficial nutrients, and it really *is* a paste, so we'll not glamorize it. Rather, let it glamorize you.

Milk of Roses really has its basis as much in almonds as roses, and the milk aspect comes from the opaque liquid produced from ground almonds and flower water. Putting the two together is creating a luxury item that cherishes your skin and brings you an extra glow.

Use your blender and make a paste by reducing a cupful

of blanched almonds to a fine powder and adding enough rose, elderflower, or orange blossom water to create a medium-thick mixture. Gradually add enough additional flower water to make a loosely flowing paste. Last, beat in a few drops of tincture of benzoin. Because benzoin is quite sticky to work with, first remove the Milk of Roses paste from the blender, and beat in the benzoin by hand. Strain and bottle for use as a tissue builder, skin invigorator and refresher.

Cucumber/Milk Summer Facial

In various travels I've made searching for practices of women who have increased their health and attractiveness through simple means, almost without exception one basic item has been repeated over and over. I have been offered dozens of differing applications involving the cucumber. In England an actress I met in a greengrocer's told me she soothed her skin after removing stage makeup by rubbing in repeated applications of cucumber juice.

A Turkish beauty I interviewed for a feature story said the cucumber was a favorite among her friends who used it to counter oily skin. In some areas of the world the cucumber has a different look and taste, but its cleansing and cooling properties remain intact. In the Netherlands, the cucumber grows nearly two feet long. A former airline stewardess from Rotterdam, who had settled down to earth in a real estate office and who helped me find an apartment, told me she used the pulped cucumber to overcome fatigued skin at the end of the day.

Probably one of the all-time favorites for summer can be found in this facial mask. The cool and tingly cucumber, which is rich in sulfur and silicon, joins forces with the calcium in powdered milk and the tightening qualities of egg white.

Cucumber Mask

Toss into the blender one-half cup of chopped cucumber, two teaspoons of powdered milk, and one egg white. Blend into a smooth paste and apply in upward swirling motions onto both face and neck. Allow the mask to dry for at least 30 minutes before rinsing away with warm water. Splash cool water onto the face and neck and blot dry.

General Care/Cucumber Milk Lotion

I am a better gatherer than I am a recorder. I don't recall where I came across the following use of the magnificent cucumber. It turned up in my file on Sumatra, when I was gathering information on the origin of benzoin, that fragrant resin that has been used in temples as an incense, in medicine for its carminative qualities, and in perfumes and facial lotions. But obviously I was intrigued with the combination of cucumber and an aromatic gum, for I've tried it and found it tightened the skin tissues slightly, and so has a place in somebody's life. Use only a thin coating and allow it to dry on the skin.

Remember, drop by drop with the benzoin. Don't be heavy handed (except in the shaking), or otherwise you will have a curdled, sticky solution on your hands (and your face, if you use it). Only a very few drops of the benzoin are needed.

Cucumber Milk Lotion

Finely mince one cucumber and cover it with boiling water. One-third cup should be enough. Cover the saucepan with a lid to prevent evaporation and simmer over very low heat for a half hour. Strain into a small bowl and add, drop by drop, enough tincture of benzoin to create a milky appearance in the cucumber liquid. Pour in one-third cup of boiling water; then pour the liquid into a small jar and shake well to blend.

General Care/Coconut Oil

It was in Panama that some youngsters shinnied up a coconut palm to get the coconuts for my hosts to show me how to prepare oil from this fruit. Incredibly agile, the two boys had me openmouthed in wonder as they ran up the slanted but towering palm, almost as though they were running into the sky.

What to do with this rich oil? In the islands they use it to give a shine to the hair, though you must be prepared for its oily quality. Coconut oil can be rubbed into the body prior to a good soaking bath, to bring suppleness to dry skin.

Coconut Oil

Drain the milk from two coconuts, and allow the coconuts to dry for a few days. Grate the meat and add one-half cup of water. Knead for several minutes to work out the residue milk. Strain into glass, porcelain or china cookware. Boil the milk without stirring for an hour to an hour and a half. Then strain the remaining oil through cheesecloth, cool it, and pour it into a bottle.

To go a step further and clarify the coconut oil, add three times as much water as there is oil. Boil the two together for about 15 minutes. Then pour into an enamel, china or porcelain basin, skim off the oil, and discard the water. You now have a fine quality coconut oil.

Oily Skin

Before attempting to cover up an oily complexion, try to discern its cause and work from that point. Check your diet and eliminate as much animal fat as possible. Also eliminate white sugar, pastries, soft drinks, fried foods, candy and all other processed foods. Construct a new diet around fresh fruits and vegetables, and their juices, plus quantities of fish, poultry and meat, or other protein sources. Add brewer's yeast to your daily diet for the invaluable B vitamins which will help normalize oily skin conditions. This regimen should go far in reducing skin oiliness.

According to Thomas H. Sternberg, M.D., in his book *More Than Skin Deep* (1970, Doubleday), excess oiliness can also stem from an endocrine or other physical cause, as well as from excessive secretion from the seborrheic (oil secreting) glands as a result of a prolonged anxiety state.

From an external approach, there are many effective ways to reduce skin oiliness: After washing your face, splash on a final rinse containing apple cider vinegar (a few drops to a glass of water). This insures removal of any soap film, and will leave you with a cleansing, oil-removing sensation. Or choose a soap with a pH compatible with your own skin.

Or you can cleanse your face with a slice of raw potato. Fresh tomatoes, too, are especially beneficial in removing oily skin wastes.

Brewer's Yeast Mask for Oily Skin

I receive many complaints from women whose skin suddenly turns oily during the summer months. One of the causes of such seasonal excesses of oil is continuing a winter diet, too laden with oils and heavy foods, instead of switching over to a lighter diet more suitable for the summer months. Daily intake of plenty of fresh fruits and vegetables should help this condition, if it is related to diet. A large salad of fresh vegetables every day, less meat, and more meat substitutes will help to clear oily skin conditions.

Brewer's Yeast Mask

A brewer's yeast mask halts the formation of excess oil on the skin, if only by cleaning the skin deeper than soap and water can reach. Try mixing a teaspoon or so of brewer's yeast with enough yogurt to make a loose, thin mixture. Pat this thoroughly into all the oily areas of the face, and allow it to dry on and remain for 15 minutes. Rinse the dried covering away with warm, then cool, water and blot dry.

Another helpful practice is to prepare a mild lotion of lemon water. Squeeze one half of a lemon into a cup of water. Instead of scrubbing your face frequently, try splashing on the lemon water and gently blotting—and removing—the surface oil. Keep a close watch on your skin to avoid irritation from the lemon water. If the solution seems too strong for your skin, add more water, or substitute skim milk for the water.

Makeup Remover for Oily Skin

"What about those of us with excessively oily skin, who use makeup, but cannot find a suitable makeup remover, or one that isn't greasy?" That's a question I hear frequently. Some readers write me that they resort to astringent lotions for makeup removal. Yet because of the usual alcohol content of such astringents, these are not suitable solutions to use daily, unless you prepare your own, minus any alcohol.

For those people with oily skin, a skim milk makeup

remover is really ideal. The drying quality of the milk seems to reduce the hyperactivity of the sebaceous glands, at least temporarily. In addition, it leaves a nourishing film on your face, instead of the remains of an inert cream.

For convenience, keep a container of powdered milk in your bathroom. Pour a teaspoon or so into a custard cup or other container, and mix with warm water to create a milky consistency. Apply with cotton balls, rub gently over all areas, then remove with facial tissues and blot dry.

Astringents

Astringents are most often used to decrease the oiliness of the face. They are excellent for this purpose as long as they don't contain alcohol. Unfortunately, most astringents do have a concentration of alcohol, which can leave the skin feeling dry and taut. So in overcoming one problem, another is created. However, you can prepare your own astringent lotion and be assured of benefits without side effects. Or search out products in health food shops that have their ingredients listed, to be sure you are not putting alcohol onto your skin every day.

No-Alcohol Astringents

Many herbs can be used as astringents; cinquefoil, witch hazel twigs, blackberry leaves, goldenrod and celandine are just a few. And they can all be obtained from an herbalist, a botanical supply house or a health food shop.

The same method of preparing a whole lemon cooked in water to be used as a hair spray (see "Treating Your Tresses") is equally good for the oily complexion. Dilute with enough water to avoid skin irritation. I keep a small jar of this creamy, lovely scented mixture beside my sink to use on my hands after contact with soap. The acid in the lemon counteracts the harmful alkalinity of the soap.

Sage used to remind me of Christmas, for that was the only time of the year it was tucked into the dressing for a roasted chicken or turkey.

But I have since become accustomed to the clean, pungent aroma wafting up from a summer hillside on an island in the Aegean Sea, a garden in Italy, and in herb patches just about everywhere. An Arabian proverb declares that a man cannot die if he has sage in his garden. Even if you are not convinced of that promise, turn to the sacred sage and lemon tea to unwind, and a splash of lotion for refreshment.

Sage Astringent

During the summer, pinch off a few leaves of fresh sage and chop them for an excellent facial astringent lotion. Drop a handful of the leaves into a cup of water. Bring them just to a simmer, then remove from the heat and let them steep until the liquid is room temperature.

Moisten your face with the liquid and feel the invigorating action, in addition to its fine cleansing power. Rub it into the summer body to soothe itching skin, and apply it to aching feet that have been confined too long in shoes.

Witch Hazel Astringent

The antiseptic quality of witch hazel adds its value as a pore tightener to this beneficial lotion. So here we are getting a two-in-one beauty treatment for oily skin by temporarily reducing the large pore size that many times accompanies oily skin.

Lemon Refresher for Oily Skin

A fine skin refresher for oily skin is made by mixing lemon juice and water, according to the strength you prefer, and freez-

ing it in an ice cube tray. As you feel the need of a refresher, remove an ice cube and run it lightly over your face. Remove both oil and moisture with cotton balls. This treatment will leave you with a cool, tingly feeling while it helps to alleviate your oily skin condition.

Facial Fruit Masks

Because of the awakening clamor for natural, untreated foods, grocers' shelves are once again becoming filled with fresh, unpreserved food items. As one consequence, instead of opening cosmetic jars and sniffing the contents and asking "What will this do for me?" we can pick up a vegetable or piece of fruit, ask that question, and receive a much more positive reply.

You've only to know your type of skin—its problems and tendencies—and the qualities of any specific fruit or vegetable, to choose the results you desire. Facial fruit masks are enormously practical. A few minutes of wearing a mask made of soft, pulpy fruit can help to correct a variety of complexion ills.

Pears and Melons

The astringent effect of a pear facial is highly desirable, especially for those with oily skin. There is also a disinfecting action, brought about by the use of a fresh, ripe pear. This would be a helpful mask for an acne condition, or any similar disturbances.

Using the juice of watermelons as a refreshing facial has long been a favorite in the South. Many claim it can remove fine-line wrinkles. It certainly offers instant stimulation. On the other hand, honeydew melons are supposed to help dry skin. These naturally purified fruit waters offer numerous benefits, not the least of which is that of cleansing and tightening soft, lax pores.

Mosaic Skin

Having a mosaic skin type means having a complexion that is not all one type or another. We speak and work so much in generalities that we can be momentarily nonplussed when we cannot apply a single solution to a single condition.

But things are not always black and white, and the in-betweens I call mosaics. Mosaics require thought and a little extra attention, if only because they cannot easily be labeled.

The unfortunate people who are afflicted with dry skin in some areas of their face, and oily skin in others often despair of successfully treating both problems. Granted, it cannot be done with a single solution, but taking the time to care for both conditions separately will pay off.

For the oily area, apply a covering made from a bit of beaten egg white and lemon juice. Rub this in lightly. Then mix a small amount of gelatin with water and rub this into the dry area. After 30 minutes, rinse both away with warm water, then dash cool water onto the face and blot dry.

Dry Skin

Some of the most annoying problems are the simplest to deal with. Dry skin is not a problem that can be solved overnight, nor can the skin be made immediately supple if it is inclined the other way. Start first with a corrected diet. Be sure you have enough polyunsaturated oils in your daily diet. Just a couple of tablespoons or so a day of an unsaturated oil can give a dry, problem skin renewed life and resiliency. And get rid of the flakes. If you use the oil in a salad, combined with lemon juice or apple cider vinegar, be sure you drink the leftover dressing in the salad bowl—it won't help your skin if it is left in the bowl.

Milk Cleanser

In addition to getting oil into your diet when you suffer from a dry skin condition, cleansing your face with whole milk instead of soap and water will help, too. Warm a couple of tablespoons of milk just slightly, add a few drops of oil and shake vigorously in a small jar to blend well. Dip cotton balls into the solution and cleanse the skin.

You will be amazed to find that it removes makeup that remains even after using a cleansing cream. In fact, for this treatment, you can skip the cleansing cream and rely solely on the milk. Use only cotton balls to apply, not paper tissues. Reserve the latter to remove both milk and makeup. Apply a thin film of oil to the skin afterwards to seal in the moisture.

Moisturizers

The cosmetic world has discovered moisturizers, and many consider this a boon to skin beauty. In today's world we are assaulted by pollutants and we spend our days in overheated homes and offices. In addition, we are addicted to the poor practice of summer tanning. Such abuses cause us to search for a preparation that will restore moisture to the body surface, while acting as a barrier to the irritating elements attacking our skin. Moisturizers are emulsions of water and oil which preserve or add to the skin's own moisture to avoid a too rapid rate of evaporation. By depositing a light film on the surface skin, a moisturizer prevents dehydration of the tissues. A moisturizer can be applied anytime to a clean face. It is especially helpful when used under your foundation or powder base.

Though there has been some question about whether the skin can be beneficially hydrated by a moisturizer, Dr. Morris Leider, Associate Professor of Dermatology at New York University School of Medicine in New York, feels that a moisturizer does that and more. By smoothing the skin and lubricating the surface, a moisturizer reduces friction.

This doctor does raise a question as to whether continual application might interfere with normal desquamation, the flaking off of dead surface cells (*American Cosmetics and Perfumery,* March, 1972).

Actually, in the area of moisturizers, I think it is everyone to her own taste. Moisturizers are really being hard-sold right now, and I've had women tell me their skin improved tremendously since using them. Some writers in the beauty field deny their value. I believe that whether moisturizers are beneficial or not depends more on the ingredients than on personal opinion. In view of the established fact that the skin can absorb a topical application, it seems to me whether you call it a moisturizer, barrier to the elements, or whatever, if there are nourishing things in the solution, then the skin can indeed benefit.

I do have doubts as to the efficacy of using commercial moisturizers whose content may include glycerin, mineral oil, and other harmful substances. To me, a moisturizer can be as uncomplicated as the application of a thin coating of oil to a face just washed in warm water, the oil applied and smoothed out with a splash of cold water and a good tissue blotting. The moistened skin tissue will plump out slightly from the warm water and the oil coating will help prevent quick evaporation of the water.

Facials for Dry Skin

When you are certain your diet is not lacking in oil, there are some facials you might try to soften your dry skin.

Apply a liberal amount of sesame seed oil to a clean, uncreamed face. Massage in gently and apply a small towel, dipped into hot water and lightly wrung out, to the face, leaving the eyes and nostrils clear. You will lie down for this one, preferably on a slant board to get the blood to your face more easily. Repeat several times, and then apply a cool, weak astringent lotion to remove any traces of oil.

You might also want to try a puree of carrot mask.

Vitamin A is more easily released in cooked carrots than in raw ones, so cook a few carrots, then drain off the water. Mash the soft, warm carrots and place between gauze and apply the gauze to the face. Leave an open space around the nose and allow the mask to remain on until it is cold. Remove and rinse the face with warm, then cool water and blot dry.

Corn Mask for Dry Skin

A fresh corn mask offers a feast to the starved complexion. This one works best if you are fortunate enough to be able to pick a tender young ear of corn fresh from its stalk.

Without wasting any time, husk the young ear and remove the silk. Run the sides of the corn down a grater. This cuts into the kernels and exposes their rich, milky fluid. Catch the grated kernels in a small bowl.

Next, gather the handful of kernels and strain them through a loose cheesecloth bag. Open the cheesecloth if necessary to allow all the pulp to get through. It is only the hulls we are trying to discard. Now, pat this milky mask onto your face and neck. Allow it to remain until it dries, or for 15 to 20 minutes.

The high protein and fat content of the corn soothes

dry skin while at the same time offering the building material needed for a healthy skin.

Those of you with dry skins are less likely to be troubled with this condition in the summer months, for then the humidity is higher and moisture loss is not as rapid. In addition, all manner of self-helps are available, and if you pay a little extra attention to your needs, you might overcome your problem.

For the days your skin is especially dry, cleanse your face with a split grape. Not only is this lubricating to the skin, but it is nourishing, and wonderfully refreshing.

The juice of wild grapes offers a wealth of valuable minerals to the skin. But your backyard may be short on this variety, so take whatever you can get in the market and give your skin a feast.

I remember so well the quick, purple-rich taste of the fox grapes we pulled each summer from the vines that bordered my grandmother's garden in Louisiana. While Grandmother checked for fresh vegetables to tuck into her basket, we children would stuff ourselves on the small, dark fruit that hung like black pearls among the tendrilled green leaves.

"Why," we asked, "are they called fox grapes?"

Grandmother would eye the forgotten hoes, the untended rows of English peas, and the neglected lettuce.

"Because the foxes who live beyond that fence happen to be partial to them."

We would peer beyond the garden into the deep woods festooned with Spanish moss and decide perhaps we would stay inside the fence for a while and not strip the vines of *all* the grapes.

In later years, though, we took a page from Grandmother's own book and instead of eating the wild fox grapes, we carefully split them and applied them to teenage complexions that were blotchy, oily or dry, or simply felt a need of this very natural, very rich, distilled beauty potion.

Grandmother's beauty advice said emerald green grapes were for dry skin and the darker varieties for oily skin. But I believe each grape has qualities good for both skin types.

Blackberry Wash for Flaky Skin

Sometimes help for our cosmetic problems is no farther away than the nearest hedgerow. When I was a child, I picked tiny buckets of plump dewberries or blackberries every so often and sold them to my mother for ten cents a bucket. I was staggered by my fortune. Little did I know that later in life I'd be picking the leaves to prepare a wonderful lotion that money cannot buy. Not only do I find the simmered brew, strained and cooled, excellent for the skin, but by using it as a final rinse for the hair after shampooing, I can cut down on the frequency of shampoos.

Flaky, problem skin can many times be helped by a tingling wash of blackberry leaves. Juliette de Bairacli Levy, one of my favorite herbalists, says in her *Herbal Handbook for Everyone* that blackberry leaves are rich in medicinal properties. She suggests that a standard brew of the leaves sweetened with honey is a cure for blood and skin disorders and also suggests applying the same liquid, minus the honey, as a treatment for eczema.

Dry Skin Caused by Harsh Weather

The assault of winter weather on delicate tissues causes problems for many women. One way to defend your skin against the ravages of harsh weather is to be sure that your winter diet has not changed radically. Include fresh fruits and vegetables in your daily diet and avoid an increase in carbohydrate consumption. Also, be sure you are getting enough unsaturated oil in your diet, for oil can do wonderful things for dry skin and hair. Take vitamin E along with the unsaturated oil to keep the oil from turning rancid in the body. Try also the Papaya Steam Facial described in this book.

An unprotected skin can suffer greatly from extreme weather conditions. A dry skin will be most harmed by lashing winter winds. I have seen whole villages of Portuguese women along the Nazaré coastline north of Lisbon with exquisite complexions, though they are out in fierce weather as they meet the fishing boats and help bring in the catch and prepare it. Their complexions seem to be completely unharmed by the pelting salt spray because their diet consists mostly of fish, and of course, they get all the rich oils from this diet to protect their skin.

If your skin is dry or average it will be to your advantage to plan a defensive campaign. Use a rich night cream which has a lanolin base, for lanolin is closely akin to the oils in the human body. Or gently massage in a thin coating of oil and lemon juice, and blot away the excess.

In addition to these measures, feed the skin during the daytime, even if it is only a bit of egg yolk and milk beaten together and kept on for 15 to 20 minutes before it is rinsed off. Then, before you go out, use a thin layer of olive oil or other soothing oil on your face. Only a small amount is necessary, and after applying it, splash on warm water and spread the oil across the face. Next, splash on cold water mixed with apple cider vinegar and very carefully pat the face dry.

If you wear makeup, the oil base can become a foundation over which you can add anything you choose. The main thing is that your skin will be protected with a thin coating of oil and an acid mantle that prevents winter flaking.

Air Conditioning Can Cause Dryness

Recently a friend who has edged into her forties announced she had had enough birthdays and would not acknowledge another until the business world changed its attitude toward maturity. So I was not surprised when in response to another friend's question about her age, she answered, "Thirty-nine and holding."

It so happens that this woman looks less than the 39 she decided to hold onto. But I am sure this is because she values her appearance and comfort, and because she has a position that requires a presentable appearance.

It was she who told me of experiencing deteriorating skin quality until she realized that one cause was the hours of exposure to air conditioning in her office and home.

Air conditioning can be the very cause of skin dryness. By extracting humidity from the air, the air conditioning unit becomes an appliance not really beneficial to skin health. The principle of air conditioning is similar to that of a refrigerator, and you know what happens to food left uncovered there. In the arid parts of the country, air conditioning units actually add moisture to the air by an evaporative process of drawing air through a moistened filter. But in other areas, moisture is removed. So protect your skin with some moisture-guard.

Dry, Irritated Skin in Middle Years

Many women go on for years with a beautiful complexion that they don't have to work to maintain, only to find that when they reach their forties, their skin begins to feel dry and is easily irritated. They have been spoiled by having naturally lovely skin, and often become impatient when problems begin to appear. If this is your situation, you should be more concerned than impatient. Skin problems seldom clear up by themselves if harmful habits continue, or if neglect is a way of life. If you are experiencing sudden complexion problems, consider the following: Have your habits changed? Were you more active as a younger person? Are you receiving the proper nutrients? Do you get enough sleep? What is your skin cleansing agent?

You can see that an undesirable skin condition is not necessarily related to just one cause. The body is a unit and must be considered as such when you try to overcome a problem. Seldom if ever can an emollient or other comforting application really correct and eliminate a skin disturbance that is caused by neglect of the body. It can prove only a palliative treatment that doesn't attack the real problem.

According to I. H. Blank, Ph.D., in an article prepared at the request of the Committee on Cutaneous Health and Cosmetics, and presented in *Cosmetics* in 1973, dry skin is often secondary to mild inflammatory reaction.

No cures were suggested in this paper, but it does seem sensible to examine your living habits and attempt to correct the problem from there. Back we go to the oft repeated suggestion that a sufficient amount of polyunsaturated fat added to your diet will help you overcome a dry skin/dry hair problem. In the meantime, you might find comfort in applying a thin coating of fresh cream to your skin. The vitamin A in raw, certified milk is a beauty potion all its own.

Suntan/Sunshield Lotion

Today's trend toward deeply tanned skin in the summer can result in dried out skin for even young, healthy people. According to Albert M. Klingman, M.D., in an article in the *Journal of the American Medical Association,* December 29, 1969, sunlight, rather than the aging process, is mainly responsible for the worst manifestations of senile skin. If your skin is drying out at an early age, then I'd say you're well on your way toward destroying it. Sun damaged skin reflects itself eventually in a leathery, non-elastic condition suggestive of a tanned hide.

Premature aging is obvious in many outdoor workers who do not shield themselves well enough from the sun's rays. In addition, overexposure to the ultraviolet rays of the sun makes one a candidate for skin cancer.

There are sun shield lotions on the market, of course, though I can't vouch for their degree of effectiveness or their safety. You might like to try a sesame seed milk lotion that is pleasant to apply and seems to modify the sun's rays.

Grind a handful of sesame seeds in the blender. Add water enough to cover and whizz until you have a milky lotion. Strain through gauze and rub the lotion into your skin before going out.

This liquid will wash off in water, so reapply it after every dip in the pool. Sesame lotion will also help you to tan evenly. And it leaves the body silky smooth without dryness after bathing.

Another sun shield lotion that's simple to make calls for equal quantities of apple cider vinegar and a good vegetable oil. Olive oil is excellent, but you can use sesame, corn, or other vegetable, seed or nut oils. Mix well and apply to the body before going out in the sun.

Suntan

In those parts of the world where the intensity of the sun can quickly sear unprotected skin, women are serious in their pursuit of soothing lotions and skin tone restorers. I would say that Spanish women are extremely knowledgeable in matters relating to the skin. Though today's woman in Spain is certainly not as confined as she once was, and enjoys a career or not, as she chooses, in earlier times she was discouraged from going anywhere alone. So during the long, hot days, she remained in her own home and courtyard. Limited in this manner, the Spanish woman would spend hours-pampering her skin, rubbing in lotions made from jasmine flowers and rose water, and avoiding the sun. But as we know, tans can be acquired by reflected sunlight. So there was great interest in removing these effects.

In the plains regions of Andalusia in southern Spain, where I was given the following recipe, the daily assault from the blazing sun makes such applications necessary. This particular preparation helps to refine and remove skin discolorations caused by overexposure to the sun.

Skin Lightening Mask

Beat together one egg white with its equivalent of fresh lemon juice, both at room temperature. Place the mixture in a custard cup in a pan of hot water over a very low flame. With an ivory or wooden spoon, stir and beat the mixture until it develops a custard consistency. Cool and apply to your freshly scrubbed face. Wear from one to two hours during the daytime, or overnight.

Suntan Lotions

For those unabashedly determined to make like an Aztec princess, even at the cost of skin health, there are a couple of preparations you might want to put together, which should provide greater sunscreening power than the usual commercial preparation. One of these formulas is from Dr. Robert Alan Franklyn of The Beauty Pavilion on Sunset Boulevard in Los Angeles. Dr. Franklyn says the most effective protection against ultraviolet radiation comes from natural creams based on natural oils, like sesame and safflower, rather than the mineral oil base used in many commercial creams.

Sun Cream

Dr. Franklyn calls his preparation Sun Cream and suggests mixing all the following ingredients in a blender until smooth:

4   ounces yogurt
6   tablespoons water dispersible lecithin
2   tablespoons sesame oil
2   tablespoons safflower oil
2   tablespoons avocado oil
2   tablespoons sunflower seed oil
3   tablespoons water
1   tablespoon potato flour

Apply before going out into the sun.

Fading Tan

Part of the price you must pay for long hours in the summer sun is a sickly, fading tan along about October. Marie Antoinette bathed suntanned areas of her body with buttermilk and apparently achieved a fine porcelain look, according to her biographers, and as shown by her portraits. As a matter of fact, she insisted her ladies-in-waiting join her at her little farm near the grand halls of Versailles Palace, and assist her in milking the cows. This stately queen seemingly enjoyed nature as much as court life, and must have been incredibly chic in the gingham gowns she and her retinue wore for their outdoor chores. She probably wasn't very much liked by the elegant court women, though, and had to listen to their wails over acquiring unfashionable tans.

So they would plaster faces, shoulders and bosoms with coatings of sour milk, in order to appear evenings in the porcelain fashion of the day. Yogurt is probably easier to apply and seems to do just as well, but it has to remain on overnight, successively, until the skin takes on a livelier, more even color.

To assist in the removal of the leftover tan, cranberry juice has proved to be of great value. The bleaching qualities of this acid fruit do much to remove the yellowish discoloration.

Fresh cranberries should be used for this. Simply crush a handful at a time in order to extract the potent liquid. Rub this into the face and neck areas, and any other part of the body you might want to treat. You might apply the juice at night and rinse it off in the morning. It is usually necessary to repeat the applications over a period of several days to achieve the desired results.

The four acids contained in the cranberry bring about the bleaching action that clears and stimulates the skin.

If the astringent action appears too strong when left on overnight, try periods of shorter application until you find the right length of time for your own complexion. You might also keep the skin well lubricated between applications of the cranberry juice.

Wild watercress can usually be found growing near small streams in the summer. In addition to being a tasty addition to warm-weather salads, the pungent leaves of the watercress can be used to make a face wash that is excellent for rough textured skin. You might want to try this watercress lotion particularly in the early fall, when a fading summer tan appears unglamorous.

Watercress Lotion

To make the watercress lotion, drop a freshly rinsed bunch of cress into two cups of cold water (spring water or mineral water is especially good), bring to a boil and simmer gently for ten minutes. Strain into a jar, and use at room temperature. Bathe both face and throat (and hands, too, for that matter) with an old piece of white towelling dipped into the liquid. Allow the lotion to dry on the skin; later rinse it away with warm and then cool water.

Facial for Sallow Skin

Women with sallow skin often find that the sallowness deepens with passing years, and their complexions lose their alive look. You cannot, of course, change the yellowish tint which gives your skin its particular color. You *can* check your diet to determine if you are receiving the nutrients you need to insure an active circulation that will carry away body wastes. Poor circulation can give a drab, muddy look to the skin. You can also help activate circulation by applying a soya powder and yogurt facial twice a week. The stimulating effect of the facial hastens the flow of blood to your face and brings new life to a weary complexion.

Mix a teaspoon of soya powder with a tablespoon of plain yogurt and blend together. Gently rub this mixture onto the face and neck areas. Allow it to dry for 30 to 40 minutes before rinsing away with warm and then cool water. Use a sturdy face cloth for the final rub, then blot the skin dry. If any dryness occurs, pat in a thin film of oil and blot again. Another aid is watermelon juice, allowed to dry on the skin.

Facial to Lighten Olive Complexion

An olive complexion may turn darker during the early summer months. If you wish to lighten an olive complexion, turn to the vegetable patch instead of to compounds containing mercury. You may find frequent applications of fresh, vine-ripened tomatoes helpful. The acid content of tomatoes makes them an excellent bleach that can help lighten the effects of the sun. Apply mashed, pulpy tomatoes to your face and neck. Rinse the pulp away when it has dried.

Pineapple Enzymatic Action for a Lifeless Complexion

A lacklustre complexion of gray tones can be the result of the wrong diet. But if your nutrition is well balanced and your skin remains dull, perhaps you need a fresh pineapple facial. This is a remarkable treatment for the wan complexion that is understimulated. The bromelain enzyme in the fresh pineapple actually dissolves the top layer of dead cells and rids your skin of this smothering blanket which prevents it from breathing, and encourages a dead tissue buildup that no cream can remove.

Fresh Pineapple Facial

If you have a juicing machine, plan for a pineapple juice cocktail, perhaps mixed with carrot juice, and reserve one fourth cup of the pineapple juice to use as a soaking facial. Saturate a double thickness of gauze in the fresh juice and, lying down, place the gauze over an unoiled and uncreamed face. Leave the moistened gauze on while you take a fifteen minute rest. If full-strength fruit juice proves too strong, you can dilute it with a small amount of water.

Rinse your face in warm water and with a dry washcloth, rub your face gently to remove the softened layer which has been loosened by the enzymatic action of the fruit juice. Easy does it to avoid irritation. Rinse again in warm and then cool water and blot dry. Next rub in the contents of a vitamin E capsule to nourish and soothe. Go to bed and forget it all and awaken fresh faced.

Apricot Mask for Dull Skin

Apricots are a valuable skin food. Try mashing to a pulpy consistency a fresh, raw apricot and patting it onto the skin that is dull and lifeless without obvious reason.

If fresh apricots aren't available, try the sun-dried ones without sulfur dioxide used as a preservative. These apricots are also beneficial to tired skin, and they bring their own bleaching qualities to the unevenly tanned complexion. The apricot mask offers something to all types of skin. But it really comes into its own in bringing enriching minerals to the anemic complexion.

Try using a mask of this fruit every other day and work toward a steady once or twice weekly apricot facial schedule. From the beginning, the frequent applications can stimulate and enliven the wan skin.

Usually the lifeless skin is also an early wrinkling skin, and frequent applications of either fresh or dried apricots will help to ease this condition.

Dried Apricot Mask

To prepare the sun-dried apricots, soak them overnight in water deep enough to cover the fruit. The following day cook them gently at low temperature until they are soft. Use no sweetening in the cooking process, though you might choose to add honey when you use the apricots as an internal food.

You will need only one or two apricots for your mask. Mash the warm stewed apricots to a soft pulp and apply a thin layer to your face and throat area, continuing around the sides of the neck. Wear the mask for ten minutes and then remove and rinse away the remainder.

End-of-Winter Masks

One of my main sources of pleasure during the years I lived in Paris was the twice-weekly *marchés,* or outdoor markets, where planked stands supported jewel-toned pyramids of fruits and vegetables which beguiled the eye and tempted the appetite.

Sometimes I didn't even get to my classes at the University because the produce enticed me to market too long, or madame the *légumière* would repeat a fine recipe for *ratatouille,* a stew of many vegetables. Or perhaps, indulging my other interest, she would relate a beauty preparation put together by her own mother, a raving beauty who would have put the legendary *femme fatale,* Ninon de L'Enclos, to shame.

And though the vegetable woman's cheeks might be touched with over-exposure to the raw weather and dampness of this part of France during the winter months, she would swear to the efficacy of all the preparations her beautiful mother put together from the abundance of nature around her. For herself, pfah! she didn't care. But her mother had gone to the grave in her ninetieth year with the complexion of a young woman. Because she was of the people, with no great means, she had relied on nature for her cosmetics. Ground and sifted eggshells for powder, beets for lip and cheek coloring, and camomile for lightening her hair.

Woods, fields and streams yielded up beauty potions to correct the cares of each season, madame informed me. Each quarter of the year produced its own problems and remedies. And what of winter, I asked? What did your mother find to overcome the deadly pall of a winter complexion? For sometimes the rain of Spain falls first in Paris for weeks running. And if one is forced to remain too long indoors, it shows on the complexion.

"Ah, ça fait une autre paire des manches," madame would exclaim. That makes another pair of sleeves—that's another story. And so it was.

Madame's clever mother would steam her face first with a dried peppermint brew to cleanse the skin, pore deep. Then while the skin was still warm she would gently massage in a solution made from an unbeaten egg white, a few drops of camphor and enough warm milk to make a loose paste. After this dried on the skin, she rinsed it away and dabbed on warm honey (heated over hot water). When the honey was sticky-dry, she rinsed it away and rubbed in a film of warm olive oil, splashed cold water over the area and blotted away all but the faintest film.

Sometimes a formula like this would constitute my lesson for the day and I would spend the remainder of my time beating up a batch of *ratatouille* for dinner and also plaster my face with the results of my belief in madame's sainted mother's approach to being a natural woman.

And if madame's moon colored eggs were in heavy supply, she would enthusiastically tell me of the sheer magic of using egg yolks beaten into water or rum for a super shampoo. I've since wondered if she hadn't gotten hold of Madame Pompadour's own handbook to beauty care. But what matter? The formulas always worked, for the fruits of nature used wisely will always have a place in any beauty regimen.

For those who are grayed from too little physical stimulation, sallow from lack of fresh fruits and vegetables, and colorless from scant sunshine and fresh air, there are additional ways to stimulate the skin and improve the blood circulation for which it has been starved.

For your end-of-the-winter pickup, you might want to try a brewer's yeast mask. It is really effective for increasing the circulation of the skin. You'll actually feel the pulling and gentle tightening of the mixture as it begins to dry on your skin.

Wheat germ makes another excellent mask for stimulating winter skin. This nutritious food, as you know, is removed during the milling process as wheat is being turned into the white flour so damaging to good health. While we should include wheat germ in our diet to regain nutrients that would otherwise be lost to us, we can also employ it in various ways externally as we work to bring out our beauty.

One such way is to use the mask for stimulating and nourishing the skin. While a brewer's yeast mask is more for normal or oily skin, wheat germ can more profitably be used by those with dry skin.

Wheat Germ Mask

To prepare the mask, place a tablespoon each of raw wheat germ and water in a clean custard cup or other small dish. Be sure you have raw wheat germ rather than a toasted, heated, or otherwise tampered with product.

Also, because the oil in this delicate food grows rancid very easily, try to find wheat germ that is vacuum packed, in order to get it at its best. Keep the jar refrigerated to prevent deterioration.

Beat the mixture until the germ grows a bit soft as it dissolves into the liquid. Now add one teaspoon of egg yolk, fertile if possible. Save the remainder for another mask by leaving it in its shell and placing it in a closed container in the refrigerator.

Beat the wheat germ, water and yolk until a fairly smooth mixture is obtained. Now apply the mixture to a clean face and neck. Pat the mixture into the skin, not missing any area. Wait a moment until it begins to dry a bit, then add more until you have a nice layer covering the entire area. Allow the mask to dry for 15 to 20 minutes.

To remove the mask, dip a fresh washcloth into a basin of warm water and apply it to the covered area. Gently move the cloth over the skin, then rinse the washcloth over and over, so that each time you return a fresh cloth to your face. After all of the particles of the mask are removed, dash cool water over your face and neck.

Poultices for Skin Impurities

Lotions and potions can be peddled and pushed for all they're worth, but when it comes to cleansing and clearing up a skin outbreak, I'll stick with the old fashioned poultices with which I was plastered on more than one occasion as a child and later as a teenager. And that's because I have a mother who knows many of the growing things that help and heal. It just would not have occurred to my mother to send to the drugstore when anyone in the family had a skin problem. Why, you just slapped on a poultice and let it draw out whatever had to be drawn out.

The Madeira vine that shaded our veranda from the summer sun was used on more than one occasion to clear up a case of adolescent problem skin. Mother would cook the fleshy white root she dug from beneath the vine, mash it pulpy, and apply it to an ailing skin.

But the house that looked out over cotton fields has long since disappeared, as has the Madeira vine that no one where I now live has ever heard of. But there is another plant with equally admirable qualities, and this weed-cum-herb is available in herbalist shops, botanical supply houses and some health food shops.

Dock is a member of the familiar sorrel family. The drying quality of dock probably accounts for much of its value as a facial pack. It's been used for centuries to treat itching skin and skin eruptions. In addition it acts as a gentle astringent tonic to the complexion.

Dock Poultice

The roots are steamed to a mashable softness, gathered between gauze squares (double thickness), and placed while still very warm on the troubled skin to draw out impurities. When the dock mash cools, replace with another filled gauze. Keep this up for half an hour or so. Don't overdo it by having the mash too hot; you can judge what is comfortable.

If you absolutely can't abide a pudding on your face, then mash the roots to a pulp and mix with the water in which they were cooked. Strain and bathe the face with this lotion several times a day until your skin has cleared. This latter method will probably take longer, but it works just as well as the poultice.

Sunflower Friction Rub

Sunflower meal is a superb rejuvenator for the complexion. While it is better to grind your own, this can be purchased already ground.

For ease of application, mix the meal with warm milk to moisten. Splash warm water across your face, and scooping up a handful of the gray mixture, gently rub it into and around the entire face and neck area. Rich in vitamins E and D, this sunshine food used as a skin rub will work its own wonders, even when used only as an abrasive.

Cornmeal as Beauty Grains

Perhaps it is my southern heritage, but corn remains one of my favorite grains, as a food and as a cosmetic aid. This golden kernel has long been appreciated in the southern part of the world as nature's health offering. The American Indians used corn as both food and medicine. Asthma, spasmodic conditions and even heart conditions were treated with various corn preparations.

The Mayas of Yucatan equally appreciated the medicinal values of corn, and relied on this staple as their main food source. On a recent trip to visit the ruins of the Mayan city of Chichén Itzá, I came across an area where huge, carved stones had formed the House of the Corn Grinders. One could imagine the continuous labor needed to grind the golden maize in the hollow stones.

Finely ground cornmeal is a superb skin and scalp cleanser. I use it frequently as a skin smoother, and especially like it as a means of preventing dead tissue buildup.

Moisten a handful of fine meal and rub into all parts of the face and throat. Be especially attentive to the area around the nostrils, for this friction scrub is excellent for combating the blackheads that often develop there.

A stay in the hospital may leave your skin muddy and dull. Antibiotics, those powerful bacteria destroyers so widely used today, cannot distinguish between good and bad bacteria. So when you take antibiotics, the intestinal flora are destroyed along with the attacking bacteria. As a result, your food probably isn't being properly digested and you may be experiencing faulty elimination. The skin serves as an organ of elimination when the conventional channels are not effective, resulting in the muddy appearance so common to hospital patients. To restore a healthy glow to your skin, start eating yogurt and other sour milk products. Increase your vitamin B intake to encourage the growth of intestinal flora. In short order you should have a much clearer complexion.

We have day faces and night faces, and woe! if we try to get through an evening with a leftover day face. That is why extra care is so very important if you don't want to appear as a ghost of yourself late in the evening hours. By day's end the skin will sag in weariness if you've had a busy time of it earning a living and solving problems. So it is up to you to remove all makeup, refresh the skin, and proceed from there.

Skin Tightener

If you are in need of a skin tightener, for those nights when your face just seems to sag, try this combination of foods. Mix together two tablespoons of egg white, one tablespoon of powdered milk, and one-half teaspoon of honey. Beat together until well blended and gently pat into all areas of the face and throat. Allow this to dry on the face and rinse away with warm water. Splash on cold water and blot dry. Finally, apply an herbal astringent (mint, sage, etc.) lotion and allow this to dry on.

Skin Cleansers

Soap is by far the most popular skin cleanser, but its alkaline quality strips the skin of its acid mantle, leaving it dry and flaky. In addition, dirt and grime can begin to collect on the skin within a short time after a soap and water scrubbing. There are some few soaps now with a pH compatible with your own. One is a bran and oatmeal mixture, another is a protein bar. But these cannot be found in a supermarket, and even many soaps in a health food shop will be alkaline. Purchase brands that clearly state their pH level. If necessity causes you to use an alkaline soap, splash on a final rinse of apple cider vinegar and water to restore your skin's acid mantle.

Many women are attracted to scented soaps because of their convenience and pleasant fragrance. But the perfumes in these bars are sometimes more irritating to the skin than the alkalinity of the soap itself. If you really wish to use a scented soap, there is an easy way to make your own.

Since soaps absorb odors so easily, you can produce your own scented bar without having the actual perfume irritate your skin.

Buy several bars of your favorite non-alkaline soap and an air-tight box to keep them in. Soak pieces of cotton or gauze in lavender or other scented oil, which you have purchased from a botanical supply house or other reputable source. Place the scented cotton or gauze around the bars of soap and leave for a month or two before using the soap.

There are many other cleansers you can use which not only deep-clean your skin, but nourish it at the same time.

Oatmeal and Cream Cleanser

The old standby of oatmeal and cream is a marvelous natural cleanser that you can whip up by yourself in just a few minutes. Grind some oatmeal (not the instant type) to a powder and mix in enough cream or milk to make a medium paste. Smooth this onto the soiled areas until any accumulation of dirt is removed. Rinse and blot dry.

Almond Meal

Almond meal is an excellent skin cleanser and smoother that has been used for centuries by women with all manner of complexion problems. It is delightful to use, and easy to prepare. Almond meal is a deep pore cleanser and once you have cleansed your skin well, any roughness should disappear.

I know almond meal was sold in this country for years, and it was probably a regular item on our mothers' and grandmothers' dressing tables. Unfortunately, it appears to have gone the way of many simple and effective beauty items, such as pure rose water, bottled only yards away from where the flowers grew, and elderflower water, the gentle and sweet liquid that was indispensable to an older generation as coverbase is to the present one.

But there really is no problem as long as you can walk into a market and buy a bag of almonds. Almond meal is one of the simplest of items to prepare. In five minutes you can have a supply of really fresh meal to last as long as you like.

Almond Meal

Take whatever quantity of almonds you choose (one-half cup, one cup, etc.), put them into a saucepan and pour boiling water over them. Let them soak until the water cools enough to loosen the skins. Slide the brown covering off the nuts and place the blanched almonds on absorbent toweling. When they are completely dry (overnight drying is best) drop them into a nut grinder, or blender and reduce to a fine powder. If you're rushed, dry the almonds slowly in the oven, then proceed to grind them.

Place a container of meal beside your wash basin and store the remainder in your refrigerator. When you are ready to use the almond meal, wet your hands and face, shake some of the meal into your hands and rub a bit more onto the face and neck area.

Rinse carefully several times in order to remove all of the meal and skin debris. You will immediately feel the smoothness of your skin after such a wash. Almond meal could permanently take the place of soap and water scrubbing for the face.

Lime juice can be used to dissolve the flaky top layer of skin on your face. Apply to a freshly washed face that has been rinsed several times in warm water to help open the pores and soften the debris. Squeeze the juice of one half of a lime into a cup of warm water and dip a washcloth into the mixture. Squeeze out the excess water and cover your face with the warm washcloth for several minutes. Remove the washcloth and rinse the face over and over in warm water. Now take a fresh washcloth and rub gently at your skin. This should remove the loosened skin and produce a fresh, shining complexion beneath. Apply a thin coating of oil to soothe the skin.

Black skin is quick to show dead tissue buildup. Though this sloughing off of lifeless tissue is quite normal, it is more apparent on dark skin. Creams and oils are of little help in overcoming the condition, for the dead cells must first be removed. A rough textured loofah mitt is helpful here if used daily.

But to overcome this ashy appearance that is usually found on the heels, knees, and elbows, use a pumice stone while bathing. Then a cream or lotion with a pH compatible with your skin can be massaged in. Or mix equal quantities of olive oil and lanolin over hot water and blend in a few drops of lemon juice, and apply daily after bathing.

Special Problems/Blackheads

While washing the face is important in controlling and eliminating various skin distresses, it is more a matter of *how* you do this, rather than how often. In addition to avoiding harmful foods, clogged pores call for a regular and thorough cleansing program. No half-way measures will eliminate the troublesome spots that can mar an otherwise attractive face.

Here's where a beauty brush or a natural sponge from the sea will come in handy. The beauty brush is the more effective of the two; it should be of natural bristles, and designed especially for the complexion.

Make a good lather of fine almond meal and water and gently work this foam over the face. The fine bristles of the brush ease into every pore to cleanse and open the clogged skin. But take care not to use the brush too energetically or you might irritate your face even more.

The skin will be naturally sensitive to this treatment the first few times, but a good almond meal and brush cleansing of the too-oily skin is an effective measure in combating blackheads.

If you don't own a complexion brush, and prefer to try the more easily available sponge, be sure it is not a plastic sponge. The porous sponge I suggest is a natural element of marine life. This type of sponge is excellent for the skin, and can replace the usual washcloth. While the brush is really preferable for eliminating blackheads and keeping the pores open and cleansed, the sponge can be used to maintain the cleanliness of the skin. Be careful to keep both brush and sponge immaculately clean.

In addition, there is an English washcloth with a slightly abrasive quality on the market. I always take mine when

I travel, for it dries overnight and does a thorough job of cleansing the skin.

Blackhead Cleanser

You will also want to try this simple-to-make blackhead cleanser for oily skin. To one-fourth cup of finely grated non-alkaline soap, add one-fourth cup of cornmeal and one-fourth cup of almond meal. Keep the mixture in a closed container beside the sink and use once or twice a day.

When you are ready to wash your face, pour a small amount of the cleanser into a custard cup and add just enough water to make a fairly loose paste. Apply the mixture to your face with a moistened brush or sponge. Lather the foam thoroughly into every pore, especially where the blackheads are concentrated. This action will help to dislodge the embedded dust and oil. Afterwards, rinse the face thoroughly in warm and then cool water. As a final rinse, use a tablespoon of apple cider vinegar to a cup of water and splash it on your face, then blot the face dry.

Many of the commercial preparations designed for enlarged pores and blackheads serve only to dry out and irritate the skin, without actually helping to solve the problem. Whenever nature in her impressive simplicity can be put to use, it seems far wiser than depending on a manufactured application that might irritate or clog pores that are already overburdened. An excellent cleanser and antiseptic lotion for oily skin and the problems this type of complexion engenders can be made from fresh, iron-rich parsley.

Place one bunch of parsley into a pot and cover it with the non-gaseous type of mineral water. Soak for 24 hours. Prepare the skin by washing it thoroughly, rinsing it with warm water and patting it dry. Soak cotton balls in the parsley solution and apply to the affected areas. In addition to cleansing oily skin, this refreshing parsley lotion will lessen redness of the skin tissues.

My last trip to Spain yielded this useful formula. I had gone into a small cosmetic shop in the clay colored city of Toledo to buy their famous cucumber cream. While I was there, a young girl came in and asked for something to cover her blemished skin. The lovely Castillian saleswoman proceeded to lecture the girl on skin care, and it was here I learned about the parsley treatment for clogged pores.

The first method was the one suggested by the Spanish woman to her client. But you can also prepare the parsley solution more quickly, the American way I suppose you could call it, since we are always looking for shortcuts.

Drop a handful of chopped fresh parsley into a cup of boiling water and let steep until it is room temperature. Apply this solution in a wet compress to the face for 10 to 15 minutes each day until the condition clears up.

In addition to external attention when dealing with pore clogging blackheads, check into your diet to be sure your vitamin A intake is sufficient. Lack of this vitamin can create dead cells below the skin surface which clog the oil glands and pores and prevent the normal lubrication of the skin. As the foreign matter remains in the pores and distends these delicate openings, large pore conditions will develop. So begin your campaign by increasing your vitamin A intake if that is necessary, and use the parsley lotion every day.

Calcium for Acne

Many dermatologists correctly consider the fact that improvement on exposure to sunlight, which helps the body to manufacture vitamin D, is proof that nutrition is an important factor in treating acne. They suggest that this vitamin, plus fresh fruits and vegetables rich in minerals, should form a part of the overall acne treatment. Yet a good proportion of the dermatologists who treat acne with vitamin D seem to have forgotten that the role of this vitamin is to facilitate the body's absorption and use of calcium. They administer the vitamin alone and wonder why it is not as effective as sunlight in the summer, when the patient is also eating plenty of fresh, calcium-rich vegetables.

An adequate intake of calcium depends on more than simply swallowing foods supposedly high in calcium. First of all, do those foods you rely on for calcium really supply your needs? Drinking milk is not sufficient in itself for those whose tissues are seriously deficient in this mineral, according to Adelle Davis.

Sunflower seeds are an excellent source of calcium and in addition, offer a vegetable source of vitamin D. Supplements of bone meal would certainly seem indicated here, in order to assure the proper amount of calcium intake. Calcium lactate is another excellent source, and a good choice for those who don't need the additional phosphorus contained in bone meal.

Burdock for Acne

While correcting the diet to include fresh fruits and vegetables, and an abundance of foods containing calcium, you might also want to use a burdock facial steaming formula that has helped many acne sufferers in their battle. Softening the hardened skin layer and bringing relief to these lesions, at the same time the astringent liquid will remove excessive oil from the skin. This weed-cum-herb has long served as a healer of poor skin conditions. But you must be patient and use the herbal liquid fully 15 minutes a day until you notice improvement.

Burdock Anti-Acne Steam

Drop a double handful of dried burdock (leaves, roots or burrs) into two cups of cold water, bring to a simmer, and retain this degree of heat for three to four minutes. Strain the liquid and place in a glass or enamel pot in which it can be reheated several times during the 15 minutes. Dip a clean, white terry cloth into the warm liquid and hold it against the affected part of the face until the heat is gone. Repeat the procedure for 15 minutes, reheating the liquid as needed in order to maintain a warm temperature.

While a burdock facial will not get rid of an acne condition, its healing and soothing properties serve to lessen the swelling and inflammation that accompany acne lesions. And used in conjunction with improved nutrition, daily exercise, enough sleep, and sufficient quantities of calcium, you may be able to help control this condition.

Taken as a tea, the burdock plant is helpful for all blood disorders, according to Juliette de Bairacli Levy. Anyone with a skin affliction could safely use the tea as a beverage, while at the same time applying the tea to the irritated area. Use one ounce of the root in three-fourths pint of water, simmer for 15 minutes and steep for three hours. Drink a small cupful sweetened with honey twice a day.

Emergency Measures

Papaya mint tea is another excellent treatment for an acne explosion. But only when used as a hot facial pack, with a cloth dipped into the brew and held to the affected areas for 15 minutes, at least twice a day. As the liquid cools, reheat to an extremely warm temperature and hold the saturated cloth (white, please, though the tea stains badly) to the face until it cools, dip and repeat.

The college daughter of a friend called in tears one day to say she had cut classes for two days due to a severe facial eruption. She had gone to a dermatologist who proceeded to open up several lesions on her face with needles or whatever those instruments of torture are. By morning my friend's face had blossomed out all over, even after taking newly prescribed medications from her doctor—so the victim refused to leave her room, saw no signs of relief, and had no desire to return to the doctor who, she felt, had "done her in," as Liza in *Pygmalion* would say. Knowing my love of and belief in herbal applications for everything from a dispirited skin to a bruised ego, she asked for a magic potion. Magic is different things to different people. My bag of tricks will always include papaya mint tea bags for emergencies.

I told her how to prepare the papaya solution; two tea bags steeped in a cup and a half of water until a strong brew emerged. Heat to the highest degree of temperature bearable to the skin and proceed to apply in a compress to the area.

By morning the eruptions had subsided and within two days her skin had resumed some degree of normalcy. This beautiful formula was suggested to me by a doctor who treated her patients solely with nature's gentlest products, and it seems never to fail. However, do not use on skin with red veins showing.

Help for Boils

Many people ask me for advice on how to care for skin that is susceptible to boils. I do not diagnose or prescribe, but because of the apparent relationship between the skin and the B vitamins, I want to share with you the findings of Dr. Katsu Takenouchi, professor of dermatology at the School of Medicine of Japan's Chiba University.

Dr. Takenouchi compared the skins of healthy patients with those of dermatitis sufferers to measure vitamin B content. He found that 27 percent of those with skin infections were deficient in thiamine, 27 percent deficient in riboflavin, and 52 percent deficient in pyridoxine. Dr. Takenouchi points out that about one percent of the vitamin B taken into the system is channeled to the skin. In order to maintain a level of one-half milligram of thiamine in the skin, you must consume 50 milligrams of thiamine.

Professor Takenouchi found the following skin diseases to be directly associated with vitamin B deficiencies: eczema, dermatitis, multiple erythema, keratosis, virus disease of the skin, skin tuberculosis, skin syphilis, baldness and various types of discolorations.

So be sure you get ample amounts of the B vitamins in your diet, from natural sources like wheat germ, brewer's yeast and desiccated liver. If you are practicing good nutrition by eating plenty of fresh fruits and vegetables, and cutting down on processed, fried and heavily seasoned foods, then your problem skin should show continued improvement.

Certain foods are especially helpful in ridding the body of accumulated toxins and cleansing the bloodstream, which helps, in turn, to keep the skin blemish-free. Cranberry juice is a most effective blood cleanser. It is rich in potassium, a mineral needed by the body to aid in disposal of waste materials.

Try drinking a glass of the juice each day. Make it a practice to have a large raw salad daily containing lots of watercress, another noted blood cleanser. Cucumbers are also excellent for the skin.

Cold Sores

Cold sores are a great problem for many of us, especially during the winter months. Called *herpes simplex* by the medical world, these painful blisters which hover around the mouth but can be found also on other body areas, are considered virus infections. Adelle Davis suggests using vitamins B$_6$ and C, plus pantothenic acid, along with highly fortified milk to combat cold sores. She describes this method of treatment in her book, *Let's Get Well.*

Keep the area well lubricated. There are some preparations on the market which help keep the fever blisters lubricated and thus alleviate some of the discomfort. Another type of preparation dries out the blisters with a minimum of discomfort.

Poison Oak

For those plagued with poison oak and similar rashes during the summer, here's a suggestion to help ease your discomfort. From Hawaii comes the practice of using the aloe vera plant growing in or around your home. A pot kept in the kitchen is a bright idea, for it proves invaluable in treating burns, too.

For poison oak, cut off a frond, remove the needles and cut in half to expose the inside. Chop into small pieces. When the egg-white type of substance is rubbed over the affected area, it will relieve the itching and promote the drying of the rash. You can keep the frond in a plastic bag and use it over and over. Moisture seems to return to the frond after it rests for awhile.

The aloe plant is now used by medical manufacturers in various cosmetic and medical products. Aolygalacturonic acid, which is a derivative of pectin and is found in the aloe vera plant, offers its healing qualities for a variety of ills. Burns, sunburns, skin eczemas, impetigo, psoriasis, skin fissures, and sebaceous skin disorders are just some of the many ailments aided by direct application of the aloe gel, or as it is produced by manufacturers in combination with a cream or unguent base. It has also been found helpful in clearing up cases of dandruff.

Fresh Vegetable Facial Masks

Carrot Mask for Blemished Skin

A preparation of raw carrots, mashed to a smooth paste, does wonders in helping to clear a pimply complexion, when it is used along with regular good nutritional practices. The high vitamin A content of this red-gold vegetable no doubt explains its helpfulness.

For the carrot mask, pat the ground vegetable over the entire face and throat area. Rest quietly, lying down, for 15 or 20 minutes. Then remove the mask and rinse off the face and neck and pat the skin dry.

Feel the smoothness that comes from this beauty treatment. Notice the cleanliness and firmness of the skin. You have actually applied a living mask, capable of imparting its own valuable and vital elements when you use fresh vegetables in such a fashion.

For the greatest benefits from such living masks, one must begin with a clean, freshly scrubbed face. This means that it is necessary to avoid a residue of cleansing cream on the skin, for this would prevent easy penetration of the vegetable juices, which should be free to touch and nourish the skin directly, rather than being separated from the pores by a barrier of oil.

If you'd prefer to use carrots in a softer form for a facial mask, try steaming them until they are tender, without seasoning, of course. Mash them to a soft pulp and pat a good covering onto the face. Relax and enjoy the warm and nourishing mask for 15 or 20 minutes. Then remove the mask, rinse the face and pat it dry. Try to add to the mask the water in which the carrots were cooked for extra mineral content.

Small whiteheads which stay under the skin are a rather common cause of distress. Not only are these little bumps unsightly, but they seem not to respond at all to any type of cosmetic treatment. They can prove a most baffling and frustrating problem, and afflict both men and women.

Since no external application helps in treating this problem, it would appear to stem from diet. Adelle Davis says that when volunteers in experiments remained on diets deficient in vitamin B_2, not only did the facial area become excessively oily, but tiny, fatty deposits appeared under the skin.

In trying to improve a lingering skin problem, it would be wise to check your diet and learn how you might be depriving your body of its needs. Because of the interaction of one B vitamin with the others, it is important when correcting such a deficiency on your own to stick to food sources that supply these B complex vitamins in the correct proportions. Wheat germ, liver and yeast are all complete sources of the vitamin B complex. If you add sufficient quantities of these foods to your daily diet, you should be able to correct your skin problem.

Those of us with a sweet tooth may have a tendency toward outbreaks of pimples. Snacking on fruits will not always satisfy a craving for sweets, and an unwise choice of snack foods often has a great deal to do with a blemished complexion. But as long as the right foods are consumed at mealtime, there is no reason to give up energy-boosting snacks between meals, if you don't have a weight problem.

Here is a recipe that will satisfy anyone's sweet tooth, and it gives you a terrific energy boost.

Sweet Tooth Energy Booster

Put through an old fashioned food grinder (the one you turn by hand), on the next to smallest cutter, one cup each of dried dates, raisins, figs, pecans, apricots, unsweetened coconut shreds, and sunflower meal.

Mix the ingredients well, and then add three tablespoons of honey and enough of your favorite fruit juice to moisten the mixture. Adjust the amounts of liquid and sunflower meal to create a mixture thick enough to form into a tight ball. Pat the ball out onto a countertop and roll the fruit mixture to a thickness of one-half inch. Cut into squares and allow the candy to "set" for several hours before eating.

Another type of skin problem that defies conventional cosmetic solutions is the outbreak of hard, dry pimples that resemble "goose bumps." The outbreaks can range from fine patches to large welt-like bumps over the arms and legs.

According to nutritionists, pores plugged with dead cells cause a skin condition that resembles goose pimples, though they are not related to heat or cold. The rough patches of dry skin affect the elbows, knees, buttocks and back of the upper arms. If the pores which are plugged with dead cells and oils become infected, pimples usually result.

Doctors and nutritionists suggest adequate intake of vitamin A to relieve and eventually clear up this condition. Fish liver oils are an excellent source of vitamin A. Liver, green leafy vegetables, apricots, carrots and sweet potatoes also provide substantial amounts of this essential nutrient.

Vitamin A requires many helpers in order to be fully utilized in the body. Both bile salts and vitamin E must be present for this vitamin to be absorbed by the tissues. And without the B vitamin choline, vitamin A cannot be stored. A balanced diet is essential in treating a disorder such as this one.

Rough Skin

Body sleekness is actually a convenience, and those little extra attentions we pay ourselves contribute to an overall sense of comfort, so necessary if we are to put self from mind in order to get on with living. A roughened skin catches at clothing and creates concern in knowing that we're not as perfect as we could be with a bit more effort.

Sifting down through cosmetic history are notations on the merits of the elderflower in soothing and smoothing distressed skin. Victoria B. was so convinced of its helpful qualities that when she escaped from her chateau in Germany prior to World War II, she had in her hastily packed overnight case only one change of clothing and a bottle of elderflower water. Her complexion at 80, when last I saw her, was much like the Dresden figures for which her native city was famous.

Throughout the years she was in this country, Victoria continued to prepare her own elderflower water. Greatly reduced in circumstances, she found her cherished blossoms in parks around her adopted city. Out would come a bag, and she would pick enough of the fragile flowers to make the lotion she felt protected her exquisite complexion.

Elderflower Lotion

To profit from Victoria's practices, place one cup of fresh or dried elderflowers and a cup of water in an enamel or glass container that has a cover. Steep for one full day before straining and mixing with one-half cup of fresh lemon juice.

This lotion, like all others, is applied after scrupulously cleansing the face, and removing any oil or cream.

Wrinkles and Lines

Idealization of the human body is achieved by taking the best care possible of all its parts, and eliminating practices that accelerate undue aging. Every maturing process has its place in the life cycle, however, and each age has its own purpose and grace.

But there is no reason to give in to unnecessary debilitation of the body. Premature wrinkling of the skin is usually indicative of excesses and neglect, and can be avoided or overcome. Without resorting to the impossible artifices and tiresome coquetries that belong to an earlier time, a mature woman can remain more youthful than her years by cherishing both body and soul as a divine gift, and by using a sensible approach to body care based on sound nutrition and simple practices.

In the process of maturing, some lining of the face is natural. A woman who reaches 30 without any ingraining of facial movement must be an expressionless person. Although all of us mature, we can slow down those wrinkles and keep our skin smooth and fresh for a long time. Dry skin is the chief cause of severe facial lines. Excessive sunlight, too, is extremely damaging to the skin and will create a leathering or drying condition.

If you are concerned about deepening facial lines, you might want to try including one or two tablespoons of salad oil in your diet each day. Oil will work wonders for raspy, dry skin and dry hair that has defied other treatments. As a safety measure, you may also want to take vitamin E to avoid the tendency of oils to turn rancid within the body.

Wrinkle Chasers

Any attempt to counteract the aging appearance of wrinkles is worthwhile when it involves improved diet, extra skin care, exercise and composure. Herbs, oils and other foods certainly have their place in pampering the skin in order to stimulate, normalize, feed and soothe.

A favorite wrinkle chaser among Egyptian women was egg white beaten with a few drops of lemon juice. Paint the face with this mixture and allow to dry thoroughly before rinsing off.

A couple of banana slices mashed to a fine puree and applied to the face and neck is also helpful in avoiding skin tautness that can lead to wrinkling. Or save a tablespoon of leftover breakfast oatmeal, mix with a few drops of salad oil and cream and gently rub into the face and neck area for several minutes. Rinse away after 30 minutes and enjoy a softer skin, and in consequence, one less prone to wrinkling. But this must become a daily practice, or at least an every-other-day habit in order to lessen the tendency to wrinkle.

Continual exposure to weather over a period of years will take its toll of the complexion. Wrinkled, leathery skin makes many women look much older than they really are. But there is hope for the outdoor buff who finds that most creams and lotions slide right off her skin. There is a remarkable cream on the market created by Dr. Benjamin Frank, a veteran researcher in the field of reversing the aging process. His cream is a biological skin normalizer made primarily from a strain of yeast rich in nucleic acids, which lessens the depth of wrinkled and lined facial tissue.

Dr. Frank has been researching and working for years to establish the fact that nucleic acids diminish the oxidative basis of aging. These acids also work in the domain of cellular repair. It is this medical doctor's belief that increased nucleic acid intake is a strong factor in prevention and treatment of cellular degeneration. Dr. Frank points out that there are other kinds of damage than oxidative, and that there are other processes involved in the cell degeneration of the aging process. But any improvement in the utilization of oxygen within the body is of value in continuation of life functions. And since nucleic acid can help increase one's vigor by energy enrichment, then it is easy to accept the fact that nucleic acids help to reverse the aging process.

According to Dr. Frank, wrinkles are reduced in depth and width by 30 percent to 60 percent generally with his cream. The tightening action of the cream reduces skin folds, which in turn smoothes and softens the skin. The face assumes a more youthful appearance.

Good food sources of nucleic acids include brewer's yeast, sardines, desiccated liver and sweetbreads.

Diet Can Cause Wrinkles

A protein deficiency can cause premature wrinkling of the skin, and many diets are based on extreme approaches that may bring on deep wrinkling. A lack of protein in the body can produce far more damaging results than early wrinkling of the skin. Since the body itself is composed largely of protein, an insufficient intake and assimilation can affect internal organs, too. If you have been on an extended reducing program, reassess your diet and add more protein if necessary.

Poor vision can be the cause of gathering lines around the outer eye areas. These striae are totally demoralizing to the average woman, and she fights them generally with expensive eye creams and lotions that enjoy booming sales at cosmetic counters. Yet, other than acting as a possible lubricant, I doubt that any of these various concoctions have ever really lessened or removed a single line. In fact, the ones I have tried seem without lubricating qualities. Mostly they seem oily and ineffective.

Undereye Cream

You might like to try the undereye cream I use from time to time. Mix together one teaspoon each of hydrolyzed protein, lemon juice and vegetable oil, and shake until thickened.

Remove (whenever you're ready) with a dab of milk.

Crow's feet cannot be completely removed without surgery, but they can be lessened. One man I know rubs his finger around the inside of a raw egg shell every time his wife serves eggs for breakfast. Then he rubs the white (pure protein) into the tiny lines spreading out from the corners of his eyes. He says that the lines have visibly lessened. Oil should always be applied afterwards, as egg white can be drying. Honey and egg white or honey and cream also help.

I have found that a brewer's yeast mask, patted in and allowed to dry fully, seems to diminish the two lines that run lengthward from the sides of the nose to the corners of the mouth. But this cannot be a hit or miss operation— dedication is required if you want to soften those lines.

Prepare a yeast mask (see index) two or three times a week, and do not rush the treatment, for the yeast, in drying, contracts and tightens the facial tissue, decreasing the depth of line. Remove the dried yeast by using warm and then cool water. Pat dry and gently rub upwards and outwards with sweet almond oil or another nut or vegetable oil, for the yeast can be drying to the skin.

Wrinkles around the mouth can have several causes,

including the habitual pursing of the lips to express a mental attitude. You may not even be conscious of what you are doing, but this act can mar an otherwise pleasant face. Pursing of the mouth can be an unconscious expression of concentration, disapproval, or similar mental states.

These creases in the skin become more pronounced with age, especially when the skin has not been properly cared for and cannot bounce back to unlined smoothness.

Here is a simple exercise for the mouth area. Make an "O" without allowing the lips to close. Try to widen the "O" without allowing the size of the lips to move from their constricted small "O." Practice several times a day.

Another exercise is to open your mouth slightly and move your lips in a clockwise direction starting at 12 o'clock, and very slowly following the imaginary hands as they move all the way around the clock until you have returned to the 12 o'clock position. Now reverse the movement and start in a counter-clockwise position. Do these exercises several times a day and you will benefit from the toning of the area.

Yet another aid in fighting mouth lines is frequent application of oil to keep the skin soft. To help the oil to penetrate, dampen a washcloth with warm water and apply it to your face to open the pores. Then, smooth on a good vegetable or nut oil. You may want to apply the warm cloth again for a minute or two, then pat in a bit more oil. Don't let it drip, and try spreading the lines gently with your fingers as you apply the oil around the mouth. Spread them horizontally, and do not use force. Pat in the oil with a smoothing motion. Try this daily for several weeks—or even months—and see if there is not an improvement. Don't expect immediate results—it took years for those lines to develop and it will take patience to help erase them.

B_{12} Can Cause Wrinkles

The tiny grooving lines above the upper lip have sometimes been associated with wearers of poorly fitting dentures. However, there are other causes. Habitual pursing of the lips can etch these longitudinal lines into catchalls for makeup and lipstick.

And prolonged use of large amounts of vitamin B_{12} many times causes a type of wrinkling, called "whistle marks," above and below the mouth. This is one of the problems that arise from isolating one of the B vitamins and taking it to the exclusion of others in the vitamin B complex. When the need for a specific B vitamin occurs, it is wise to get it from natural sources of vitamin B such as liver, wheat germ, yeast and yogurt. Continued use of one specific B vitamin increases the need of all the other B vitamins, and if they are not supplied as a unit, other deficiencies may develop. So be sure to balance your diet with vitamin B-rich foods.

Freckles

In times past, when women discovered they could not totally, or sometimes even partially, remove freckles from their skin, they developed charming names for these spots as a consolatory acceptance, and blamed iron in the blood and the light of the sun for the mischief. Some of the world's greatest beauties exhibited the distinctive spots.

Freckles usually disappear as people mature. However, in most cases a few remain to become an annoyance, and people try all kinds of lighteners to get rid of them. Generally you can fade freckles a bit with vegetable bleaches (don't try anything stronger) or conceal them to a degree with makeup. But banish them completely—never!

Other than being considered a cosmetic nuisance, freckles are disregarded by dermatologists. They are considered to be small accumulations of unevenly distributed pigment. Exposure to sunlight deepens the color of these spots.

To lessen the reddish coloring of freckles a bit, you might want to apply yogurt to them each day. Or you can crush cranberries (fresh) and rub this juice into the freckled skin. Lemon juice is another harmless bleach. This should be applied to the freckles only, using a fine camel's hair brush, both night and morning. If stinging or irritation occurs, discontinue the applications, rinse and apply a soothing film of vegetable oil to the face.

Vitiligo

Another skin aberration occurs in vitiligo, a loss of skin pigmentation which manifests itself in small white marks that appear on some areas of the body, while other areas become darker. Some nutritionists consider vitiligo a dietary deficiency. Adelle Davis recommends the use of either pantothenic acid or PABA, in addition to applying a PABA ointment to the area. Her suggestion is to increase dietary intake of all the B vitamins from natural sources. This would include liver, brewer's yeast, wheat germ, cheese and meats.

Tiny skin protuberances on the neck can be very unattractive. Some women report success with using castor oil to remove these bits of excess flesh. However, a doctor can freeze them briefly and clip them off, painlessly, in his office.

One suggestion for a do-it-yourself removal which is harmless and sometimes successful requires placing a corn pad over the skin-tag with the latter uncovered and centered in the open ring of the pad. With an eye dropper, squeeze a drop or two of castor oil onto the skin-tag and gently massage the oil in. The corn pad will prevent the oil from dripping and also prevents it from rubbing off onto clothing or bed linens.

Brown splotches on the skin are one possible side effect of taking the Pill. Though not everyone reacts negatively to this contraceptive, which has been prescribed by some doctors as a treatment for acne, many women do develop this "mask of pregnancy" as it was called in earlier days. Effectiveness of the Pill as a contraceptive lies in the fact that it produces the symptoms of a false pregnancy. This same condition of influencing body hormones sometimes will help clear up acne. But it can also bring on the mottled mantling of the skin, which, in a natural pregnancy, usually disappears after childbirth. Where the body remains in a constant state of "false pregnancy," the mask seems to remain also.

It is a sad thing to see vibrant young complexions blazoned with dull markings of bilious coloring. Yet this condition is prevalent among young women today, and only a hefty covering of makeup can conceal the mottled complexion. And for those who endure the condition for the sake of convenience, I cannot help wondering how they can jeopardize romance, and lessen the impact of an exciting perfume and seductive gown.

If you've stopped taking the Pill, the brown splotching will probably clear up after a period of time, though this is not always the case.

Generally we think of fair skin as being a desirable type, and the fragile and delicate appearance of such can indeed be lovely. But not when laced with minute red lines that wander across the cheeks and nose.

Telangiectases, as these lines are called, may be visible on the face as a network of tiny red veins that no makeup can completely conceal. These small ruptured capillaries stem from vitamin deficiencies, and can be treated most effectively by turning to nutrition as a means of strengthening the damaged blood vessels. X-ray treatments, which have been used to treat acne, can also cause telangiectases. The rays destroy vitamins C and P (the bioflavonoids), render capillary walls extremely fragile, and the blood supply is allowed to seep out of the veins into the surrounding area. Some dermatologists seal off the broken and damaged vessels with an electric needle. But whatever method you decide on, it would be wise to work also from within, to build up the blood vessels in order to avoid continued damage.

Vitamin C is found abundantly in fresh fruits and vegetables; vitamin P has a rich source in buckwheat (you can also purchase the vitamin in concentrated form, as a buckwheat derivative), parsley, cabbage, oranges, lemon juice, apricots and grapefruit, among other fruits and vegetables.

While increasing your intake of these foods internally, you might want to rub parsley juice into the affected areas several times a day. If it proves irritating, mix a bit of honey with the juice and use that.

A complexion brush used too vigorously could also damage fragile capillaries in the facial tissues. Normally a complexion brush is kinder to the skin than even a washcloth for it avoids any pulling on the skin.

Mature Skin

The mature skin should be treated exactly the way a younger skin is treated, only more so. In fact, a mature skin condition, that is, an older looking skin, can be delayed indefinitely if one starts early enough with good skin care.

There is no blanket, regimented formula or method of taking care of the skin because of age. All depends on its condition.

As a pick-up lotion, you could make an elderflower lotion (see Index), or rub the juice from a tangerine or apple onto your skin for a refreshing lift.

I once knew a woman in Italy who began to prepare her daughter for maturity at the age of ten. When her daughter reached that age, she cleared a place on her own dressing table and placed some toilette articles there for the interested girl. Mostly, she said, the items were for cleansing. A finely ground almond meal, a stiff little brush for the nails, a brush for the hair, and a flower lotion, with no alcohol content, for the face. This mother determined to give her daughter a priceless gift; a regard for her own person.

At one time court-plaster was used on the aging skin to iron it out or unpleat the wrinkles. Plastic surgery is the modern approach for an all-out attack. But each time you apply some nourishing food to the skin, you are waging your own private battle, and if you persist, the results will become visible. And because not everyone can afford costly plastic surgery, nor cares to undergo it, daily applications of fresh fruits, vegetables, oils, milk, herbs and other nutrients can be your best ally against unnecessary and unwanted aging signs.

Skin Firming Lotion

A pleasant, non-discernible lotion to use on the mature face is one made from benzoin. For this lotion, mix one-fourth teaspoon tincture of benzoin in one-fourth cup of rose water, elderflower water, or orange flower water, and strain through gauze. Apply only the thinnest covering to the face with a cotton ball, and allow the liquid to dry on the skin. Use the lotion as a face wash to firm the skin or keep it firm.

Though benzoin has been used for centuries as an incense

in the temples of the Far East, clever women learned early of its cosmetic value. While its firming qualities are known, ancient beauty formulas specified its efficiency in "calling the blood to the surface, and imparting a rosy glow." The above formula was considered useful in overcoming pallor. I use this solution when I want to apply a beneficial tightening action, and don't want an obvious application. This solution keeps well, but unless you plan to use it frequently, cut the quantity in half, or even a quarter of the amount stated in the recipe.

Always avoid an overly-made-up appearance, especially as you get older. Cosmetics applied as a cover-up can cause an aging appearance in themselves. On the stage, a mature or aging appearance is achieved with a matte finish. Youth can be achieved or enhanced by a glossy finish. Use only those cosmetics your skin requires. If you apply a powder base, try spraying a fine mist of mineral water over your face and throat area and allowing it to dry. Also, if you use such a base, be sure to apply a good moisturizer first. Another way to give a more natural appearance when using a powder base is to begin by applying a thin film of oil to the face. Next, splash hot water over the area and rub in gently, and follow this with a splash of cold water. Blot the skin dry before applying your makeup.

There is a certain moment when applied makeup looks just right. And it is *not* immediately after applying. Usually, according to the action of the skin, it is within one or two hours after application. Spraying the face after applying makeup, and blotting lightly, will set your makeup instantly.

The application of powder to the black skin can many times pose a problem because of the flat look that powder leaves on this color of skin. Though black cosmetics now include face powders of varied hues and translucence, the problem still remains for some. A damp sponge patted lightly across the face after the powder has been applied, and has set, will give a fresh, natural appearance.

Dolly, who was one of Billy Rose's Diamond Horseshoe Girls, led a fabulous life after she married a handsome Bagdadian and went to live in his fairy-tale country. This lively woman, who still practices a strict beauty regimen, gave me a wonderful tip on how to overcome a made-up appearance. Dolly is a beautiful Texas woman who cherishes her dewy, natural look. She applies her makeup and then takes a bath, keeping water off her face but allowing the moisture from her tub to soften and subdue cosmetic applications.

The Young Complexion

Many young people, with their fresh, blooming complexions, have no need of cosmetics to conceal, but desire something to keep their skin looking fresh. Cosmetics include preparations for cleansing and conditioning as well as for decorating. And some of the old fashioned preparations allow you to keep your skin in good condition without using makeup at all.

Elderflower water can help clear the complexion, hydrate the skin and normalize the acid balance. Or mix a half teaspoon of raw honey with enough mineral water to make a non-sticky lotion. Apply daily to the face and throat areas. You might also try squeezing a teaspoon of fresh grapefruit juice into the palms and gently massaging it into the skin. Or use a segment of fresh orange for this cleansing, stimulating lotion.

A tiny bit of apple juice freshens and brightens the complexion when rubbed in thoroughly and allowed to dry.

Facial Saunas

Facial saunas are a subject of some debate among beauty experts. Many people use and enjoy them. They are supposedly helpful when herbs are used in the steam. However, an official spokesman for the American Medical Association's Committee on Cosmetics and Cutaneous Health said his organization had reports from some dermatologists of evidence that the electric saunas cause jungle acne, a disorder brought on by the presence of excess moisture in the skin.

It seems to me that these appliances have their place in a beauty regimen, but must be used wisely, and not constantly. However, the sauna effect can be achieved by utilizing the steam from an open pot (being careful not to burn your skin with too-hot steam), or with hot towel packs.

These treatments are not considered safe where broken thread veins are present.

Facial Masks

There is hardly anything of a nutritious nature in your kitchen that will not add a measure of beauty and a treasure of nutrients to your complexion. For centuries, women have created masks of millet grain, wheat flour, oatmeal, and anything else that promoted good health.

According to the materials used, facial masks can bleach, tone, invigorate, clean, refresh, create coloring in the face, help remove oily debris, and add suppleness.

To improve your skin condition, you can apply a facial as often as you like. In my own work of experimenting and testing, I sometimes have three or more facials in one day. Since the ingredients in the facials are always foods, or powders like Fuller's Earth, which is, after all, only soil, my skin profits from all this attention. While the average woman may not have the time or the inclination for such practices, she still should consider a daily facial of some sort. Perhaps only a dabbing of honey on her face to soften it; or yogurt to bleach; or oil to lubricate.

Fuller's Earth makes an excellent facial mask, but it is really best for oily or normal skin. Avoid the entire eye area when applying it, and after rinsing it away, pat a thin film of salad oil into the skin, as this mask is quite drying. Most pharmacies can special order the unbleached Fuller's Earth if you request it.

Fuller's Earth Mask

One of my readers has a unique method of preparing a Fuller's Earth mask, which she finds quite successful. Mix enough earth and mint flavored mouthwash in a glass jar to create an easy spreading consistency. The mint mouthwash helps the earth to keep, and gives one a cool feeling. Apply this mixture to the face and allow it to dry before rinsing it away. Afterward, use a moisturizer. This facial efficiently removes dead skin cells and other debris. If your mouthwash has artificial coloring and alcohol, skip it and instead use mineral water or brew your own mint water.

Aromatic Vinegars

Women in less complicated times developed specialities in aromatic vinegars, and much as today's woman sometimes chooses to be associated with a particular perfume, the fastidious woman of yesterday might well have been known for her particular aromatic vinegar. Even today in Europe you can find bottles with sprigs of herbal or floral sprays immersed in the vinegar contents.

You might wish to experiment with one or two aromatic

vinegars and go on from there. It is a great deal of fun to produce your own scented vinegar water if you have discovered the benefits it gives your skin.

In the springtime, violet petals can be added to your vinegar. In summer, try the stronger scented plants. Roses, of course, are always good. Lavender flowers, honeysuckle, carnations or any of the spicy flowers add their particular sweetness to these solutions. For herbal fragrances, use rosemary, dill, thyme, sweet basil, or a combination of these or others. Any pungently scented herb will do wonders in disguising the acrid vinegar odor.

Try adding two cups of petals, or snippets of leaves, to the contents of one pint bottle of white vinegar, which has first been slightly heated. Pour the warmed vinegar over the petals or leaves and mix together in a lidded container (glass is best). Leave the solution for two weeks, and open to test the strength of the scent. Strain the liquid into a glass bottle and use, diluted, as a facial rinse that helps to fight oily skin.

Estrogen Creams

Every so often a cosmetic that catches at a woman's hopes for producing a more youthful appearance is made available to the consuming public. Estrogen cream is one such item and I can well understand its attraction for anyone experiencing the aging of skin tissues. The theory behind a hormone cream is that it will plump up sagging skin and lessen wrinkling.

Estrogen or progesterone when added to facial creams is supposed to encourage water retention in the facial tissues when rubbed into the skin, thereby creating a smoother, more filled-out face.

But according to the Delaney Committee which reported to the Eighty-second Congress back in 1953, estrogenic hormones may cause undesirable physical changes. Estrogens are absorbed through the skin, and there is variance of thought among medical men concerning the appropriate amounts to be administered. Because the hormone creams are drawn into the skin, they can cause an imbalance in the body's own hormones. There are far safer ways to maintain youthful skin.

Cocoa Butter

It is enormously comforting to find a product that has never faltered in its performance, and in its user's appreciation of its qualities. Cocoa butter, or oil theobroma, is such a product. Women around the world have delighted in this pleasantly scented and buttery soft pomade for centuries.

I was once a guest of a beautiful Trinidadian woman, in Port of Spain, whose only skin treatment was cocoa butter, applied morning and night. Her skin, at 45, was as youthful appearing and supple as that of a woman half her age. She said since she had grown up on a cocoa plantation, as had members of her family before her, she had learned to use cocoa butter for skin irritations due to dryness, and, having nothing else readily available, as a cosmetic cream for the complexion.

Cocoa butter is an excellent skin emollient, and a marvelous natural beauty aid. The oil, from which the butter is made, is obtained by grinding roasted cacao beans and separating the vegetable fat from the product we know as chocolate.

Cocoa butter is very softening to the skin, and some women apply it to the stomach and breast area during pregnancy to avoid stretch marks. It can also be used to advantage on the forehead where wrinkles tend to develop, and around the mouth to soften the lines forming there. Cocoa butter melts at body temperature, and is thus easy to apply.

Vanishing Cream

As a beauty editor, and one who is deeply interested in any and all beauty preparations, I do admit that I am occasionally mystified by a cosmetic. Such a one is vanishing cream. This dubious combination of ingredients more than ever confirms my very strong feelings about the necessity of labeling all products used in and on the body.

Vanishing cream was quite popular in past years, despite its drying effect on the skin. Made from stearic acid and partially saponified with alkali, when applied to the face, this cream combines with the mineral salts present in the skin to form a type of soap. Naturally this clogs the pores and creates dry skin problems. In addition, by wearing this covering all day, or night, the natural acid mantle of the skin is removed, and the alkaline deposit of vanishing cream can be harmful for the skin, not only in creating dryness, but in exposing it to attacks by bacteria.

Vitamin E in Cosmetics

Is there a single cosmetic application that can truly halt, or at least stymie, the sometimes rapid aging process? I know of no miracle pill or cream, but I am a firm believer in a wisely planned intake of natural vitamin supplements, and the use of some vitamins as topical applications to deter premature lining of the face. Vitamin E is at the top of my list as a supplemental beauty aid. I include it in facials and night creams, in addition to applying it fresh from the capsule to any irritation that might arise.

Many manufacturers are now including vitamin E in their cosmetics, and making claims for its qualities as a beautifying agent.

Vitamin E promotes oxygen conservation within the body, and is required for normal tissue metabolism. By helping to insure a youthful bloodstream, vitamin E can certainly qualify as a beauty vitamin, when we keep in mind that there must be good health before there can be beauty.

Since it can be absorbed through the skin, and because of its beneficial effects, vitamin E is an excellent addition to a cosmetic cream. You can create your own vitamin E cream, and probably save money, by adding the contents of a pierced capsule to your favorite cream. Many women find it helpful to apply the vitamin directly to the skin, gently massaging it in as it is applied.

Though some claims of vitamin E have been disputed, two researchers, Drs. Lester Packer and James R. Smith of the University of California's Berkeley Laboratory say they have found vitamin E capable of halting the normal aging process of human lung cells in test tubes. Vitamin E works to protect body cell deterioration. Doctors Packer and Smith confirmed that human lung cells survived twice their normal life span when vitamin E was added to the test tubes.

Lecithin

Lecithin, found in every body cell, could be regarded along with other essential nutrients as a requisite for beauty. As a natural emulsifier of fat, lecithin has the ability to assure utilization of vitamins A, D, and E within the body. I have greatly increased the effectiveness of various face and throat creams I prepare by adding a dash of liquid lecithin to the mixtures. Its equivalent would be found in egg yolks, which are beautifying agents in themselves, but don't keep as well in a skin cream.

In the diet it can have a beneficial effect on the skin by guarding against eczemas and by helping to keep the skin soft.

This fat burner is found in unrefined vegetable oils, beef, eggs, nuts, and wheat germ. A convenient method of adding lecithin to your diet is to use the granules, made from soybean oil. You can sprinkle a couple of tablespoons over your morning cereal, add it to a daily salad, or put it in soup.

Mineral Oil

The more involved I become with researching the related roles of beauty and health, the more I am turned off by manufacturers whose primary concern is one of profit from a product. It seems to me that a woman should thoroughly immerse herself in a study of harmful—and beneficial—skin applications before she buys so much as one product. I recall one manufacturer who asked my guidance in selecting an oil for a cosmetic product. His chemist had suggested mineral oil and I explained why he should not use this oil in his product. The chemist, however, informed him that he could not make as great a profit by using another oil, so the manufacturer succumbed to the persuasive chemist.

Mineral oil is widely used in commercial cosmetic products. It also appears in many recipes for homemade cosmetics, and is included in some diet regimens aimed at weight loss. The danger in using mineral oil as a food is belief in the theory that because it is not nutritious, it is not fattening or otherwise harmful. The fact is that mineral oil, a crude oil by-product, leaches out vitamins and minerals from the body when taken as a food or used as a laxative. It has also been reported as a carcinogen, or cancer causing agent.

When mineral oil is included in cosmetics, as is the case with many commercial creams, it is not absorbed by the pores but remains on the skin clogging the delicate openings and actually doing harm in its drying quality. There is certainly no merit in making your own cosmetics if you use harmful or worthless ingredients. Substitute a vegetable or nut oil for the mineral oil and treat your skin to a wealth of nutrients that will actually penetrate the pores and nourish the skin.

Medicated Soaps

I do not understand America's obsession to have medicated cosmetics, soaps, talcums, and the like. Medicated against what? Are we all so ill that we prime ourselves for battle even when washing our hands, applying makeup, or dusting our bodies for a sense of refreshment? It seems so very foolish to me to go into armed defense when there isn't even an enemy in sight. Why do consumers feel they must buy products for which there is no real need? Medicated over-the-counter or down from-the-shelf supermarket items have no place in the average life.

Various ingredients in medicated acne soaps cause allergic reactions in many people who come in contact with them. These specially formulated soaps, then, can actually do more harm than good in some cases. The Academy of Dermatology considers the antibacterial soaps enough of a hazard that in 1966 the organization suggested to the FDA the use of warning labels to explain that they have a sensitizing effect on some people—and that exposure to the sun after using these soaps may cause skin eruptions.

Lipstick

Women in earlier times probably were far more appealing and attractive, insofar as the appearance of the lips was concerned. Have you ever noticed the percentage of women whose lips are peeling and caked with lipstick? This is seldom the fault of the person so afflicted. The sufferer is guilty of nothing other than purchasing a lipstick whose ingredients have attacked her lips.

Sensitizing ingredients in lipsticks can cause the lips to react to sunlight and become irritated, which in turn can make them crack and even bleed. I have had complaints that some of the so-called hypoallergenic lipsticks do not alleviate the condition; that on the contrary, they contribute to it with their own ingredients.

The safest lipsticks I have found on the market come from health food shops. They don't wear well, but appear safe, and there is an attractive range of colors.

Black women sometimes complain about a variance in their lip color. The upper lip may be darker than the lower, or vice versa. This, they say, makes it difficult to apply lipstick to give an even appearance. There are cosmetics on the market now which meet these problems with the use of toners applied under lipsticks. Or use a pale beige undercoat of foundation before applying lipstick.

Chapped Lips

Wearing lipstick lessens the chance of lip chapping because the lips are protected from cold weather, which can be very drying. I am referring, of course, to a lipstick that doesn't cause its own damage. There are colorless chapsticks on the market, or you can make your own lip pomade of soothing, silky ingredients which will prevent chapped lips, and help to heal those already chapped.

Soothing Lip Balm

Melt over hot water one and one-half ounces of beeswax, and then blend in one ounce of honey. Beat in two ounces of unsaturated vegetable or nut oil and remove from the heat. Stir until the mixture cools and pour it into little jars. Apply to the lips before going outdoors.

The original formula used spermaceti along with the beeswax, but because of my personal feeling about endangering the sperm whale from which the spermaceti is taken, I've increased the amount of beeswax and eliminated the spermaceti. If the pomade proves a bit too hard, add enough oil to give you the consistency you want and reheat the mixture.

Lip Gloss

Personal Lip Gloss

If you prefer not to wear lipstick, you will probably enjoy making your own lip gloss. Melt together over hot water one tablespoon of beeswax and five tablespoons of vegetable or nut oil. Divide the mixture equally into three small glass jars. Into the first one thoroughly mix one-fourth teaspoon of alkanet root. Into the second one scoop out the remains of a leftover lipstick and blend. Leave the third one clear. Alkanet root produces a lovely deep burgundy gloss. It is advisable to strain this one through gauze to remove the bits of herbal coloring matter.

Chapter 2

Treating Your Tresses

If you treat it kindly, your hair can truly be your "crowning glory." Present day practices of rolling, bleaching and dyeing serve only to torment the hair of many women today. As a result, much time and money must be spent to overcome the deleterious effects of using popular commercial hair products.

Modern woman has come a long way over the ages but her hair problems have increased. Intricacies of coiffures in centuries gone by made shampooing a twice-yearly event. Although hair should certainly be washed more than twice a year, shampooing every night seems an extreme approach to its management, even in our polluted world of today.

Fads come and go, but good nutrition is still a prime requirement for maintaining a healthy head of hair. Since hair is composed of 97 percent protein, and three percent minerals and ash, a protein-rich diet goes a long way in promoting beautiful hair. Healthy hair also needs phosphoric acid, calcium, and the B vitamins. Riboflavin and vitamin A stimulate growth, and the unsaturated fatty acids help to keep hair strands from falling out.

Each strand of hair grows from a tiny indentation in

the skin called a follicle. At the base of each follicle is tissue containing blood vessels that bring nourishment to the hair shaft.

As hair grows, the old hair moves up the inside of the follicle, leaving behind a column of cells that will form a new strand of hair. As long as the old hairs deposit these strings of cells inside the follicles, the overall rate of new growth will keep pace with the number of hairs being lost. When old hair leaves the follicle without depositing new cells, it will not be replaced, and a thinning or balding process begins.

Human hair is naturally acidic. On a pH scale of 14, in which an acid state is 1, neutral is 7, and alkaline is 14, hair should register between 4.5 and 4.7. Washing the hair with an alkaline shampoo disrupts this acid balance, and can be damaging to healthy hair.

I learned this lesson early, from a classmate. Mary was a lovely girl from a Mediterranean country and she had the beautiful blue-black hair of that region. It made all her friends, including me, starkly envious. We begged for her shampoo secret, for when I was a teenager we felt that the answer to a good head of hair came out of the shampoo bottle.

But Mary disclosed that she used a bar of yellow laundry soap; the old floor scrubbing type. She said it cleansed her hair so well that she had never used anything else.

I don't know how many of our friends eventually lost their hair as a result of this "beauty secret," but fortunately my mother found me scrubbing away one day. My hair was a mass of lovely thick suds. They were doing a smashing job of cleansing my hair, but hadn't done a thing so far, to promote its health. If I continued this harsh cleansing and stripping of the hair oils, my mother informed me, I could expect to end up with strawlike hair, if any at all.

She proceeded to whip up an egg shampoo to help me overcome the squeaky clean condition of my hair. And that is when I also found out that squeaky clean isn't the most desirable clean. Whether Mary kept her hair I can't say, for we lost touch through the years, but I do know her way was not mine. Her thick masses of hair might have been able to stand abusive treatments my own fine hair could not.

How to Shampoo

Everybody knows that clean hair is important not only to help you look your best, but to make you feel good, too. For most of us, shampooing our hair is second nature—something we do once or twice a week and rarely give much thought to. But a shampoo should be planned, just as any important body care practice should be planned. Careful shampooing will keep your hair shiny and more manageable than a lot of costly creme rinses and conditioners.

Before shampooing, massage the hair by gently pulling on each strand to invigorate the scalp. Take time to do a good job and to create a relaxed feeling in the scalp area. Next, brush the hair with a soft or medium bristle brush (to avoid any irritation to the scalp that might be caused by a firmer bristled brush). Lower your head and brush from the nape of the neck upward. Cover all areas of the scalp in order to remove dust and dead scalp tissue.

Rinse the hair under a spray attachment or by pouring warm water over it. Pour a small amount of shampoo into one hand and work this into the scalp with gently rotating fingertips. Con-

tinue massaging in the shampoo, moving through the different sections of the scalp.

When you have covered the entire scalp area, rinse with warm water, holding the spray attachment with one hand and massaging with the fingers of the other. Reapply shampoo and this time concentrate on cleansing the hair strands. Rinse the hair again, using your fingertips to work through the hair and expose it to the spray. When all traces of shampoo are removed, squeeze out excess water from the hair and towel dry.

When Should You Shampoo?

How often to shampoo is a great point of contention, but it is strictly an individual matter. Generally speaking, the better your health, the less frequently a shampoo is needed. For hygienic reasons, removal of air pollutants, general comfort and freedom from unpleasant scalp odors, once a week is indicated. The timetable varies, of course, according to your particular type of hair. Is it oily or dry? Fragile or sturdy? Are you exposed to industrial air and heavy city traffic, or do you live in the comparative cleanliness of country air?

Many teenagers shampoo too often because of overly active sebaceous glands. Attention should first be given to a corrective diet to clear up this problem, and to avoid excessive shampooing that will damage the hair. If you can see comb marks in your hair after combing, that's one sign that you need a shampoo! But don't rely on this alone.

For those with dry hair, frequent shampoos can be damaging. On the other hand, oily hair calls for more frequent shampoos if it is to be manageable. Hair that is extremely dry, or excessively oily, and the scalp that quickly develops an unpleasant odor—these conditions all seem to stem from nutritional deficiencies. Until the internal requirements are met, there are bound to be difficulties in clearing up problems. At the same time, scrupulously clean hair and an odor-free scalp can be achieved by judicious use of shampoos whose frequency is dictated by need rather than rule.

If your diet is balanced and includes lots of fresh fruits and vegetables and protein, and if you have no trouble eliminating body wastes, then you should examine the manner in which you shampoo your hair, if you are experiencing problems.

A quick soaping and rinsing is never adequate for healthy hair, and in time, such short-cut methods can lead to heavy dandruff, scalp odor and clogged pores. It is far better to adopt a relaxed attitude about shampooing and learn not to depend on a quick soaping and rinsing under the shower to bring about a healthy scalp condition.

There is an old, favored recipe for cleansing the scalp that has brought satisfaction to women who had long masses of hair that could not possibly be shampooed frequently without great inconvenience.

This recipe calls for cutting a fresh lime in two, and as you need it, cutting off thin slices to reach more juice surface. Using one half at a time until it is used up, each night rub the lime surface over the scalp, without squeezing out the juice. Do not use the treatment if there are irritated areas on the skin.

Use this as an in-between cleanser, but try to avoid rubbing it into the hair itself, as it can be a little sticky to the touch. When you are ready to shampoo, use your favorite, but avoid perfumed or scented solutions. Remember, there is nothing wrong with shampooing often enough to keep the scalp clean. A clean scalp is resistant to disease.

A major selling point for many of the commercial detergent shampoos is their ability to get hair "squeaky clean." The sort of advertising that promotes squeaky clean as a desirable hair condition is misleading. We don't want our hair to squeak, any more than we like to hear a door hinge make this sound. Both conditions suggest a need for oil, or in the case of hair, a definite *loss* of oil. Hair should be supple, soft, and *silent* when it is in good condition. Detergent shampoos will indeed make your hair squeak, but at the cost of stripping the hair of all its oils.

Check your diet to make sure you're not overloading on the wrong foods. Then choose a shampoo, or make one, that is cleansing but not destructive.

Natural Shampoos

My own shampoo preferences include one made of fresh eggs, and alternately, a natural organic herbal shampoo with a pH of 4.5. It is made from rosemary leaves, mountain graperoot, soap bark, oil and lemon juice. Mine is already prepared, and comes from Canada. However, you might like to make your own, using similar ingredients.

Soap Bark Shampoo

Simmer four ounces of soap bark chips in one pint of water until the liquid is reduced to one half pint. Add a few drops of oil of rosemary for dark hair, or camomile for blonde, and blend thoroughly. This makes enough for several shampoos.

The bark from this soap tree plant contains saponin, which is capable of producing a soapy lather. The shampoo cleanses quite well without a mass of foam, and leaves the hair free of film.

Castile Shampoo

To make a delightful castile shampoo, you will need half a cup of high-quality soap made with olive oil, two pints of distilled water and one ounce of rosemary leaves.

Place the rosemary in a porcelain, glass or stainless steel pot. Pour in the boiling distilled water, and simmer gently for 15 minutes. Strain, then return the liquid to the pot and add the castile soap, cut in slivers. Heat slowly just until the soap dissolves. This may not be a highly sudsy shampoo, but it is cleansing and refreshing, and the rosemary gives it an acceptable pH.

Don't Use Soap on Your Hair

In this age of the five-minute shower, many people are shampooing their hair with the same bar of soap they use to wash their bodies. The usual bar of soap is very damaging to the hair, because it leaves an insoluble alkaline film on the scalp, even after the hair has been thoroughly rinsed. This deposit can clog the hair and oil openings in your scalp and its drying qualities help to create dandruff. In addition, the alkaline quality of soap removes the natural acid mantle of the healthy scalp and invites bacterial invasion of the area. Instead of soap, choose an herbal or egg shampoo, for a healthier scalp and better hair condition.

If you've been using soap or a harsh detergent shampoo on your hair, chances are your "crowning glory" has become limp and dried out. There is a splendid shampoo you can make at home to bring new life to dry hair. I consider it superior to any other I've found. It is my own humble version of an excellent shampoo I discovered in Paris, and loved, but no longer have access to.

Lanolin Shampoo for Dry Hair

Beat one-half teaspoon of lanolin, one teaspoon of vegetable oil, and one tablespoon of water together over boiling water. When thoroughly melted and blended together, beat in two tablespoons of herbal shampoo. If you find this mixture too soapy, the next time add a bit more lanolin and oil, in small quantities, or reduce the amount of shampoo to one tablespoon.

Rinse the hair well and add a splash of apple cider vinegar or lemon juice to your final rinse water.

Dry Shampoos

Excessive shampooing can weaken fragile hair, but you can stretch out the time between washings with a dry shampoo. You can prepare excellent dry shampoos which are quite easy to use. Finely ground cornmeal can be sprinkled through the hair and brushed out as you stand in the bath tub, or better yet, outdoors. In addition to being an effective dry shampoo, cornmeal can help clear up persistent and damaging dandruff. According to a report by L. Edward Gaul, M.D., of Evansville, Indiana, one patient whose seborrhea and hair loss did not respond to any medicated lotion used only cornmeal for a period of several months. There was a slow, but steady improvement in her scalp condition and at the end of a year, the heavy scaling, greasy scalp, and marked thinning of the hair were reversed. A medium gauge comb was suggested by the doctor for removing the cornmeal, but you may prefer a soft-bristle brush.

Use one-half cup of stone-ground cornmeal, and massage this through both scalp and hair for five to ten minutes, as required.

Bran, oatmeal and almond meal also make excellent dry shampoos.

Colorants

Good nutrition and retaining one's natural hair color seem inextricably bound together. Although there is no one formula that will guarantee the return of one's original hair color after it has faded, there are breakthroughs in the field of nutrition which give us hope that eventually we can avoid fading or complete loss of color merely by consuming enough of the right foods. Actually, there are many persons who have experienced a complete reversal of the graying syndrome by changing their diets.

While some who have used the nutritional method to regain hair color have enjoyed good results, in other cases the hair color doesn't seem to be affected at all. This is probably due to a lack of knowledge of individual dietary needs.

It is interesting to note that foods important to hair and scalp health contain the nutrients that encourage growth and prevent aging throughout the body. Nutritionist Adelle Davis stressed the need for a balance of all nutrients to insure healthy hair. This would suggest that isolating a specific type of food and using it to the exclusion of others would hardly do the trick. Rather, those specific foods that contribute especially to hair and scalp health should be used daily by adding them to an already well-planned diet.

Foods that have been found helpful in renewing faded hair color include brewer's yeast, liver, wheat germ, blackstrap molasses, sunflower seeds, whole grain cereals, rice polish, seafood, kelp, yogurt, and cold pressed vegetable and nut oils. These foods would have to be included in a regular balanced diet to be most effective.

A secondary method of combating the onslaught of fading color is to use natural colorings on the hair. Some of these can restore a measure of the original shade. Others will at least darken hair that is graying. One can even prepare a rinse from golden headed flowers that will lighten blonde hair and another herbal rinse to remove drabness.

While these colorings from herbs and flowers can help to return hair to a darker or lighter shade, they are never as concealing as chemical dyes. They can also be washed out or lightened with successive shampoos. So herbal treatments must be used on a frequent basis. This is a general rule, though of course there will be exceptions.

Hair tinting in itself is certainly not a modern innovation. It has been practiced from earliest times; probably since the day woman first became conscious of her gray hairs and associated them with a loss of youth.

Egyptian women spent hours under a kohl pack, tinting their hair as deep a shade of black as the Nile at midnight. For those who chose variety, the leaves of the henna bush were stewed to produce a bright auburn tint. Roman ladies of court used lysimachia, or purple willow-herb, to produce a blonde tint. Greek valerian, also called Jacob's ladder, when boiled in oil produced a suitable black dye. St. John's wort was counted on by the medieval English to produce a black dye capable of concealing gray hair.

Especially for Blondes

There are several old fashioned methods of returning light—and life—to darkening blonde hair. If you have that problem one of these might be of help to you.

Camomile is a blonde's best friend. This flowery, sweet-scented herb can be made into an infusion that will remove the drabness from light shades of hair, and return highlights to blonde hair that has deepened in color. Brown streaking that may come from exposure to sunlight can be minimized with a weekly camomile rinse.

Camomile Rinse

To prepare the rinse, drop a handful of dried camomile flowers in two cups of water and simmer for a half hour. Steep until warm, and strain. After shampooing and rinsing the hair in clear water, towel dry, and begin pouring the camomile solution over the hair. Catch the brew in a basin and pour through the hair several times. Towel dry again.

A different shampoo that is used for lightening blonde hair requires beating the whites of two eggs until as stiff as possible. Having brushed your hair until it is free of dust and dandruff, rub the stiffly beaten egg white into the scalp and hair a handful at a time. Use a light, circular movement of the fingers for applying the whites. Dry your hair in the sun for 20 minutes, then brush thoroughly for several minutes.

Another hair lightener is the juice of a lemon squeezed into the final rinse water after shampooing the hair. This lemon rinse should be poured over the hair several times for the greatest benefits.

Yet another favored method of restoring life to drab hair is to use ale.

Without using soap at all, the hair is washed in a warm (room temperature) basin of light ale, every other week.

It is necessary to note that you may be doomed to disappointment if you apply these simple, natural colorants expecting the same chemical sudsing, foaming, instant coloring you might get from a commercial product. And not every suggestion is suitable for every individual, but every one is safe. You must be willing to experiment to find out what is best for your own needs, since the field of natural beauty is highly personal.

Especially for Brunettes

Perhaps the oldest and best known of the several natural preparations that can add color to dark hair is made from henna, a shrub that grows in the Near East. It is dried and ground to a dark brown powder which coats the hair without penetration, and thus is considered a safe vegetable dye. The color of the hair deepens with the length of time the moist preparation is left on.

Be sure you choose a pure, powdered henna rather than a metallic compound. Pure henna, when used without a modifying agent will yield a brilliant orange-red shade difficult for many to wear. But a half and half mixture of camomile and henna will bring varying tones of reddish gold to your hair. If your hair is white, gray or blonde, don't use straight henna unless you're ready for a very bizarre color!

Auburn Tint

For a more subtle shade, add one-half cup of dried sage to one pint of boiling water and steep overnight. Then mix one teaspoon of ground cloves with one tablespoon of henna. Add enough of the sage tea to make a paste and stir until it is smooth. Shampoo the hair and rinse thoroughly. Next, towel dry and apply the paste to all parts of the hair. Comb through to insure an even distribution of color. Cover the head with an old towel and allow the color to develop for 30 minutes, or longer for a deeper shade. Rinse the hair well in warm water. This treatment is supposed to give a reddish brown tint, but can vary greatly, according to hair texture, previous color, and the condition of your hair. Be sure to make a patch test first.

The hulls of walnuts and butternuts have been used to obtain a rich, dark brown dye. It is not an easy method, but offers a source of organic color that cannot cause harm, unless you are allergic to a specific plant. For such a dye, press the juice from the green hulls of black walnuts into a jar. These hulls can be gathered in the summertime before the nuts begin to harden or dry. They have to be carefully knocked or pried off the walnut. Some herbalist shops and health food stores carry them, in case you can't locate a black walnut tree growing nearby.

Rich Walnut Tint

Add a small quantity of rectified alcohol and a little powdered allspice or cloves to the walnut juice. Place a lid on the jar and allow the mixture to soak for seven or eight days. Shake the jar several times while it is steeping. Filter through a linen cloth and add a little salt as a preservative. Keep in a cool place.

For another harmless hair dye, mix four parts of the juice of green walnuts with one part neats-foot oil, according to the amount of natural oil present in the hair. If your hair is unusually dry, you might want to add a bit more oil, and if it is oily, a bit less.

Black walnut hulls stain anything they touch, so if you intend to extract the juice, use rubber gloves, or be prepared to have stains on your hands that soap and water will not wash off immediately. Walnut juice must also be carefully applied to the hair. Otherwise you will have a darker than usual scalp.

Sage was used as a hair colorant even before it became a favorite in ancient herb gardens. This versatile plant provides a harmless and effective method of darkening gray hair. There are dozens of ways suggested to use sage to produce a dark brown shade.

Sage Tint

One of the simplest ways is to toss two tablespoons of dried sage and two tablespoons of black tea into a pint of boiling water. Cover and simmer for 25 minutes, then steep for several hours and strain the brew. Rub a bit of this liquid into the hair and scalp every day, to gradually darken the hair. When the desired shade of brown is reached, reduce the daily application to twice weekly, or less, as needed.

The sage tea must be prepared fresh weekly. If the amount suggested proves too much for a week's supply, adjust the ingredients accordingly.

Tag alder bark is another botanical brew that has been in use for some time. It is supposed to bring gray hair to a light shade of brown.

One does not often hear about tag alder bark, but if you are willing to experiment with a harmless herbal coloring agent, simmer one ounce of tag alder chips in a quart of water for one hour. Allow the liquid to cool and shampoo your hair with the liquid once or twice a month, using the quart of colorant for both shampoo and rinse.

When experimenting with these natural dyes, remember that as a woman gets older, she should not wear a hair color darker than her natural color was before it began to gray. This will age her appearance, as will dark foundation lotions and lipsticks. If your natural hair color is brown, stick to the shade most like your own.

Reconditioning Over-Dyed Hair

I often receive complaints from women whose hair has been damaged by years of stripping, bleaching and dyeing. These treatments can dry out hair to such an extent that it will not respond even to expensive conditioners, especially when the abuse continues. This type of situation reminds me of the story of the miser who taught his horse not to eat. The man was successful, but the horse starved to death. You cannot expect to continue to expose your hair to harsh, damaging conditions without having it collapse on you. Some people can get by for years with stripping, bleaching and dyeing because of perhaps 1) a good diet 2) extra hair care and 3) a sturdy head of hair.

But eventually, even the strongest hair submits to the brutal stripping and bleaching process, and whether you can resurrect it after this obvious deterioration has begun is anyone's guess. It becomes apparent that your hair is rebelling, and you must decide whether to continue bleaching and accept the consequences of eventually causing permanent damage to your hair.

When these conditions exist, I would suggest allowing your hair to return to its normal color (it really is not too difficult a decision to make: whether to have gray hair or to become bald). But for some immediate results, I would recommend a thorough reconditioning of the hair with some rich food products. First, though it may darken your hair, you could try a warm castor oil pack.

Heat enough of this thick oil to rub generously into your entire hair and scalp area. To insure the proper coating, gently comb through the strands several times. Place a plastic bag over the scalp and tuck in the sides to create as much scalp heat as possible and help in the saturation. Leave the scalp pack on for an hour before shampooing away with an herbal shampoo. Two shampoos are usually necessary to remove the excess oil. Rinse thoroughly and add a couple of teaspoons of apple cider vinegar to a quart of water as a rinse, then rinse that out with clear, warm water and dry the hair without any heat.

The next shampoo should be made of two beaten eggs, or the yolks of two eggs beaten into one-eighth cup of water. Carefully massage into the hair and leave on for 30 minutes before rinsing out without additional shampoo. Towel dry and rub in some thick mayonnaise. Use homemade mayonnaise or add an egg yolk to a good commercial brand. The homemade will be superior, because you will know what kind of oil you are using.

Massage the mayonnaise into the hair and leave on for an hour before lightly shampooing with an herbal shampoo. Rinse with a couple of teaspoons of apple cider vinegar or lemon juice added to the water. Then rinse again with clear water. This treatment will darken blonde hair, but it helps repair the damage.

Mayonnaise Conditioner

Since mayonnaise is an important part of this restorative process, it is best to make your own to be assured of high quality. Place one egg, two tablespoons of lemon juice or apple cider vinegar, and a sprinkling of salt into the blender container. Pour in one-fourth cup of cold pressed vegetable oil. Cover the blender container and whizz on a fast speed until thick and well blended. Remove the center cap from the lid and very, very slowly, pour in a thin strand three-fourths cup more of the vegetable oil while the blender is running.

Hydrolyzed protein is preferred by some people as a hair treatment because it is more quickly absorbed by the hair strands. This pre-digested form of protein is fairly expensive, but it is worth the price if you value the resurrection or maintenance of your hair. I have never hesitated to try an item recommended for good body care, even if it meant cutting down expenses in some other area. In the long run, a healthy and beautiful body is a bargain at any price!

Dry Hair

What does dry, raspy hair that defies every hair conditioner you've tried suggest? Suppleness, which can disappear when there are insufficient amounts of oils in the diet, is missing here. If allowed to remain in this extremely fragile state, the hair ends will begin to split. Dandruff or dry flaking of the scalp can also commence.

Dry hair complaints are many, and some readers of my column write me they have noticed vast improvement in their dry hair—and skin—after taking two or three tablespoons of unprocessed vegetable, seed or nut oil every day. Increasing your vitamin E intake may also help. Other readers report good results with their hair after taking cod-liver oil for several weeks.

Some women believe that oils should be eliminated from the diet in order to lose weight. But many nutritionists will be quick to tell you that sufficient oils in the diet can help you to maintain a desired weight level. When the body lacks the essential fatty acids found in oils, it must change sugar into fat at a faster rate. It would certainly be worthwhile to include a tablespoon or so of salad oil in your diet each day to bring more bounce and shine to your hair.

If you apply all the rules of good nutrition, you should begin to see great improvement in the state of your hair. At the same time, by tending to the external needs of your hair, you can increase the benefits.

Many sufferers try to subdue their dry, flyaway locks by using creme rinses after shampooing. But these rinses can cause their own problems if they are overused. Frequent applications can result in limp, hard-to-set hair. They can even damage the eyes if used undiluted. Very few users bother to read instructions stating the need to avoid concentrated applications.

While traveling in South America recently I met a woman whose hair was brilliantly black and who had a glow of vibrancy about her that comes from taking good care of herself. One beauty practice this charming South American woman shared with me was the use of pureed avocado to keep hair glossy and manageable. The avocado is an excellent source of protein and as such can nourish rebellious hair strands.

Avocado Conditioner

For this treatment, massage a finely mashed avocado into the hair and scalp for a full five minutes. Cover the hair with a plastic bag, tucking in the ends to create scalp heat, for one hour before shampooing out with a non-alkaline shampoo. Add two teaspoons of lemon juice (for blondes) or two teaspoons of apple cider vinegar (for brunettes) to a quart of water for the next to last rinse. Towel dry.

An enriched protein shampoo is also helpful to dry hair. Beat two egg yolks in one-fourth cup of warm, not hot, water. Beat together and massage into the scalp. Rinse out thoroughly with warm water.

Some women are unlucky enough to have to deal with dry hair and oily skin at the same time. It may sound like an impossible task to treat both conditions simultaneously, but there is hope.

With this combination of problems, diet would be the first place to begin corrective action. Above all, do not resort to harsh measures for treating the oily skin. Avoid lotions containing alcohol, and cosmetic preparations promising to "dry up" the oiliness. Instead, add fresh fruit and vegetables to your diet, whole grain cereals and adequate amounts of protein from lean meats, eggs, fish and poultry.

Apply cleansing, astringent facials of fresh, pulped tomatoes which are allowed to remain on the face for 10 to 15 minutes. Make up a sage or mint lotion by steeping a handful of the herb in a cup of water and straining. Rub gently into the skin while the lotion is warm, and allow it to dry on the skin, without blotting.

Next, try the honey and olive oil treatment described in "Shimmer and Shine Hair Gloss." Don't use setting gels or sprays on your hair. Brush daily, with long, slow strokes, covering all areas of the scalp.

Protein Conditioner

Shampoo your hair with an egg yolk solution, made from two egg yolks beaten into one-fourth cup of warm (not hot) water. Leave this mixture on the hair for 30 minutes to one hour, when time permits, to allow it to soak in as much as possible. Cover the scalp with a plastic bag to generate scalp heat and aid in penetration. Shampoo out by running lukewarm (never hot) water over the hair and rubbing briskly as with a regular shampoo. Do *not* use soap, or any other shampoo. This shampoo will lather beautifully. Rinse thoroughly to eliminate all traces of egg odor.

Oily Hair

Each strand of hair we see protruding from the scalp has its base firmly encased within the follicle, or scalp opening, which also contains an opening from the seba-ceous gland. This oil gland supplies a lubricant for both hair shaft and skin. And it is the sometimes overly pro-ductive sebaceous gland which can wreak havoc on the hair and skin.

Under normal conditions the sebum, or oil, supplied by this particular gland keeps the hair supple and poses no problem. But overactivity in the scalp area can help bring about the excessive oiliness contributory to sebaceous or oily dandruff, which in turn can be a step toward baldness.

There is practically no information available on causes of excessive oil secretion in the scalp area. It is possible that too-frequent shampoos can over stimulate the oil glands. Diet is a factor here, too. All I can suggest is to develop a "hair growing" regimen which concentrates on the B vitamins, plus all other essentials for super health. Such a diet plan should help you to overcome oily—or dry—hair problems, and many other scalp distresses that defy external treatment.

Controlling and Conditioning Your Hair

Keeping fine hair in place is always a challenge. Com-mercial sprays do the job, but the lacquer leaves a stiff coating on the hair, and inhaling the fumes may damage the lungs. If your hair is difficult to control, try a natural alternative to those harsh chemical aerosols.

Lemon Hair Spray

An old fashioned lemon juice spray makes a quite ade-quate "hair holder." Either use fresh lemon juice (it takes longer to dry) or cut up a whole lemon, add just enough water to cover, cook until the lemon is tender and put it in the blender. Whir until the lemon is chopped up, then strain through sufficient gauze to remove all pieces so that you are left with the liquid. Put into a spray bottle and use sparingly—it will begin to feel tacky if allowed to build up.

Use of creme rinses is not advisable when you have soft textured hair. I am personally suspicious of any less-than-natural application that takes away body from the hair.

Recently at a hearing before the Federal Trade Commission when that agency challenged advertising claims, a well known company admitted that although they advertised that their balsam hair rinse could be used as frequently as desired, this did not really imply it would be harmless to do so (UPI: December 16, 1974).

Setting Lotions

There are some excellent hair setting lotions you can whip up in no time to keep the curls in your fine hair. Try mixing one tablespoon of quince seed in one-half cup of cold water and simmering until thickened. Strain and use after cooling. This will keep for a week in the refrigerator. You can use gum tragacanth or gum arabic in the same manner.

A botanical supply house or herbalist's shop should stock these items.

Another setting lotion you might try is an old fashioned mixture of flaxseed and water. This gelatin-like solution cannot damage your hair and will produce needed body.

Simmer two tablespoons of flaxseed in one cup of water until dissolved. Strain and use.

Damp-Weather Curl Protectors

Damp weather can flatten out anyone's hair—even hair that's normally easy to curl. To keep your hair bouncy on rainy days, you might like to try one of the following preparations.

Probably one of the finest damp-weather curl protectors for dark hair is rosemary, made into an infusion and used to set the hair. Not only does it give body to thin hair, it also maintains curl throughout a damp day.

To brew the infusion, toss a handful of dried rosemary into a cup or so of cold water. Simmer for five or ten minutes, according to the strength of brew you want. Remove from the heat and steep until warm; strain and apply to the hair.

For light hair, you might try skim milk lotion, conveniently made from skim milk powder.

Try a teaspoon of milk powder to one-half cup of warm water. Increase the amount of skim milk if you require a stiffer set.

Shimmer and Shine Hair Gloss

To give dark hair a pure gloss, nothing works better than a Queen Anne's honey and olive oil pack. In a half-pint jar, pour one cup of raw honey, one-half cup of olive oil and two tablespoons of lemon juice. Place a lid on the jar and shake vigorously. If you have time, allow this to "ripen" for a day or two, or at least overnight. Keep at room temperature, and when ready to use, carefully massage into your hair before shampooing. Rub into the scalp and roots of the hair, and then comb from the scalp to the ends of the hair with a wide-toothed comb. Massage once again. Place a plastic bag over the hair and tuck in the ends to help generate scalp heat.

For quicker results, wring out hot towels and place them over the plastic bag. Repeat several times. Then allow the mixture to soak into the hair strands for a minimum of 30 minutes. Wash your hair with an herbal shampoo.

Add a little apple cider vinegar or lemon juice to your final rinse water; towel dry. Use as frequently as required.

Hair Dressings

Normal, healthy hair occasionally requires some sort of dressing to hold it in place. In earlier years, hair oils were quite popular. But applying too much oil to the hair can dull its natural lustre, especially if the hair is not dry. When the body, and consequently the scalp, is healthy, the sebaceous glands supply the hair with sufficient oils to keep it supple. Brushing can often do more for the hair than oil.

However, the following olive oil hair dressing comes from an old fashioned household manual, and can take the place of the commercial hair oils that used to be available.

Olive Hair Dressing

Mix three ounces of olive oil, one drop of lavender and one teaspoon oil of nutmeg. Heat together over boiling water until well blended. Bottle and use sparingly.

Or to eliminate the need of an external application, add a few drops of wheat germ oil to your shampoo (pour into a separate container only enough for each shampoo and mix well), and proceed as usual.

Warm linseed oil applied to the hair prior to a thorough shampooing can do an incredible "softening" job on stiff, unmanageable hair.

Be sure you purchase your linseed oil from a health food shop, or pharmacy, instead of a hardware store, for you want the edible oil rather than the type used in painting.

Conditioners

Ours is the age of bleaches, blow dryers and do-it-yourself permanents. It is also the age of the burnt-out look. But there are quick and easy conditioners you can make yourself to rescue your tormented hair.

Molasses, oddly enough, can do great things to hair that has been damaged with chemicals and otherwise mistreated. Use it as a pack for dark hair; substitute raw, light honey for lighter shades.

As another treatment (the same one suggested for damaged hair), massage in generous quantities of high quality mayonnaise to which you've added an egg yolk and a teaspoon of apple cider vinegar or lemon juice. Allow this mixture to remain on your hair and scalp as long as is convenient (30 minutes to an hour) and shampoo away. Your hair should be more supple after one or more of these treatments. Use weekly as long as your hair requires this attention.

Hair Straighteners

I receive many requests for information on hair straighteners. It seems that none of us is ever satisfied—those of us with straight hair would like it to be curly, and those with natural curls want to straighten them.

I know of no perfectly safe hair straightener. Some of them have caused balding or toxic reactions, and it is never a good idea to use chemicals to force your hair to do something it does not naturally do.

However, realizing that the desire for straight hair is just as important to some people as a permanent is to others, I will pass on the following information.

According to Dr. Irwin I. Lubowe, dermatologist at the Metropolitan Hospital Center and Flower Fifth Avenue Hospital in New York City, chemists have been testing a hair-straightening preparation being used successfully in France and South Africa. This preparation contains thiolactic acid in place of the usual thioglycolic acid, and causes less toxic reaction. Formulated by a French biologist and cosmetic chemist, the product is available in France, but not yet in the United States. This is all the news I have on the product at this time. You might check with your hairdresser for further information.

Teasing the hair in order to add height or to achieve an Afro look puts serious stress on the hair shafts, and will eventually break them. And if a straightening process has been employed previous to severe teasing, the strands are further weakened.

Dr. Algie C. Brown of Emory University in Atlanta suggests, for hair and scalp health, that black hair should be worn in its natural style. The daily insult of teasing, he points out, has been responsible for the problems of the two dozen patients he has treated for nearly complete hair loss.

Hair Sprays

In recent years, lacquer hair sprays have been among the most popular products for keeping hair in place. Now however, women are turning away from hair sprays because of their potential to harm the body. The FDA asked for recalls of hair sprays containing vinyl chloride, a propellant used in numerous commercially available brands. The recalls were spurred by the discovery that over 100 industrial workers exposed to vinyl chloride developed a rare liver cancer.

In addition, synthetic resins in hair sprays can accumulate in the lungs and lymph nodes, and are thought to be responsible for a change in lung tissue that is observable during chest surgery or autopsy. There are supposedly safe hair sprays in health food shops, but be sure to read the labels carefully before you purchase one.

Dandruff

Dandruff can begin as a mere inconvenience, but neglecting the condition in its early mild stages can ultimately have you going from one medicated shampoo to another, or from one dermatologist to another in search of a cure that could have been more easily effected if it had been started when you noticed the first flakes.

According to popular advertising on the subject, you become a social outcast when you are found with white flakes on your shoulders. Dandruff is not a pleasant affliction and probably does arouse distaste in those who see it lying in generous dustings on your blue suit or black dress. But more important, severe dandruff is an indication that all is not well with your scalp, and that its cause goes deeper than the surface of your head.

However, let's understand the difference between natural skin sloughing and dandruff, the scalp disease which affects at least 70 percent of all Americans.

Instant panic upon seeing those white flakes is many times without cause. As new cells continually form in the lower layers of skin, the outer skin at the same time is shedding or flaking, in a self disposal system. Flaking of surface tissue occurs over all the body, but daily friction from clothing and from using a towel after bathing removes these dead cells, unseen. However, the hair doesn't receive this daily friction and in consequence, brushing or combing can cause a shower of white flakes.

Other causes of flaking are hair sprays, setting gels, and shampooing liquids and soaps that have not been sufficiently rinsed out. It is only when the flaking becomes heavy, or changes in color from white to a yellowish, oily appearance that there is real cause for concern.

What you and I know as dandruff is divided into two or more types by the medical profession. And if you really want to overcome this blight you should understand the major difference between them.

The most frequently occurring of the flaking scalp conditions is called pityriasis. This dry, scaly condition comes from a natural process of desquamation, or flaking off of dead cells. Brushing the hair clean each day will usually take care of this common dandruff. However, if the scalp is irritated or itchy, brushing should be avoided.

When itching accompanies dandruff, the tendency to scratch the scalp results in irritation, which eventually produces a red and thickened scalp. Reflecting the restricted oil flow, scalp hair in pityriasis is unusually dry. Left untreated, this form of dandruff can spread beyond the scalp to infect both face and neck.

You can readily see that it is vital to avoid irritating this area, and to avoid even the use of a brush that might scratch the scalp and spread the infection. As a matter of fact, many so-called dandruff cures are chemical insults to the skin of the scalp, says Dr. Bernard Idson, of Dome Chemicals in New York City. He refers to alcoholic lotions, among others, with which a woman may douse her hair in hopes of removing excessive scaling.

Standard dandruff removers and controllers are losing favor with many dermatologists. The old sulfur solutions, resorcinol, crude tars and salicylic acid, possess sensitization potential and cause allergic reactions. And of course, hexachlorophene, the much touted dandruff chaser, has its own history of warnings to the public about its harmful effects.

However, even newer solutions should be suspect when

there are numerous chemicals tossed into the brew. A staggering amount of scalp and hair damage occurs through the indiscriminate use of so-called "miracle" dandruff cures.

Seborrheic dermatitis, the more severe type of dandruff, erupts in areas where the sebaceous glands are over productive. Too frequent shampooing can aggravate this condition. The greasy, scaly scalp, once irritated by harsh cleansers and cures, can become highly infected by bacteria. Seborrheic dermatitis is generally recognized as an inflammatory condition of the scalp.

Once you determine the seriousness of the dandruff you have, that is, if a regular shampoo and daily brushing don't minimize the fall, and if itching and changed scalp conditions accompany the disturbance, then it is time to get serious. But not by rushing out to search for a cure in a patent medicated lotion or shampoo.

Irwin I. Lubowe, M.D., professor and dermatologist at the Metropolitan Hospital Center in New York, suggests diet as the principal cause of seborrhea or dandruff of the scalp. This doctor blames the scalp disorder on faulty diet, emotional tension, infection, and injury to the scalp.

If you have a dandruff problem, the first place to start corrective action is in your diet. Cut out refined sugar and down on animal fats. Eliminate *all* soft drinks, coffee and tea, other than herbal teas, from your diet. Good hair growth can be encouraged by adding some important foods to your diet. Frequent serving of liver, to supply the B vitamins usually lacking in severe dandruff cases, is basic. Or use desiccated liver powder or tablets. These go down more easily when dissolved in tomato juice. Use brewer's yeast, cod liver oil, bone meal, vegetable oils in place of butter or animal fats, lecithin, and wheat germ. Add these to a diet rich in fresh fruits and vegetables and protein.

Anti-Dandruff Shampoo

An egg yolk shampoo has helped many people to combat dandruff. Beat the yolks of two eggs in a quarter cup of warm water, and massage this liquid into the scalp and hair for five to ten minutes. Rinse carefully and then use a final rinse of a teaspoon or so of apple cider vinegar mixed in water. Towel dry your hair. This homey formula will bring relief, and in some cases completely clear up dandruff. To remain free of this affliction, though, you must correct the cause.

Damaged Hair

Split ends are one of the most widespread hair problems afflicting women today. The high incidence of split ends can be related to excessive tampering with the hair. Bleaching, dyeing, tinting, and too-frequent use of dryers and curlers all carry their own risk.

Each hair is composed of three separate layers; the outer layer, or cuticle, has been compared to the scales of a fish, in microscopic studies. The middle, or cortex, layer is more pliable and is responsible for the color of your hair. The innermost layer of each strand, the medulla, is the receiver of nutrition. Any damage from alcohol-based lotions, sprays, or other chemicals will separate these three distinct parts. Split ends should be trimmed from the hair to avoid further separation of the layers.

Split End Treatment

Use the same egg shampoo that is so beneficial as a cleanser, anti-dandruff treatment and conditioner. At another time, apply a hair pack of honey and olive oil for badly split ends. Then wash with an herbal shampoo.

Hair is often weakened by prolonged exposure to water,

especially chemically treated water like the chlorinated water in swimming pools. Weakened hair will break easily, often snapping off halfway down its length. An improved diet will help to strengthen the hair, but external help is also needed.

Serious hair breakage among blacks should first be examined from a dietary stance. Dry, poorly nourished hair with no elasticity usually reflects a lack of fats and protein. While soul foods may be adequate in fat, they generally contain a negligible amount of protein. If your diet is limited, be sure it includes enough protein foods.

Hair Strengthener

Castor oil is one of the finest strengtheners for weakened hair.

To give your hair a castor oil treatment, rub the thick oil into both scalp and hair. Comb through the hair to insure complete distribution. Place a plastic bag over the scalp, making sure to tuck in all your hair, and leave on for an hour before shampooing out. You can shorten the time by placing hot, moist towels over the oil-treated hair. Shampoo afterwards; you may require two shampoos. Use an apple cider or lemon rinse.

Remember that no matter how much you improve your diet, and no matter what you apply externally, the chlorinated water in pools will eventually damage your hair. Wear a close-fitting bathing cap when you swim. Some instructors suggest buying a piece of chamois skin and cutting a strip to fit around the edges of your scalp, just below the hairline, inside of the cap.

Stimulating Growth

A few minutes a day spent gently stroking the hair with a natural bristle brush is like putting money in the bank;

it can be drawn on later because of the increased health its stimulation brings to the scalp.

Many women shy away from brushing the hair because of the misconception that it worsens an oily scalp. On the contrary, brushing in long strokes merely brings to the surface the oil coating the base of the hair and lying on the surface of the scalp. By more evenly distributing this output from the sebaceous glands, you can prevent eventual pore clogging and the formation of severe dandruff.

In order to avoid a too heavy deposit of oil when brushing, work a strip of gauze onto the bristles. This slight covering will absorb any excess oil. In fact, the combined accomplishments of stimulating and cleansing the scalp should leave your hair glossy and more manageable.

Use only natural bristles for brushing the hair. One of the causes advanced by dermatologists for the recent increase in balding and hair loss in women is the use of nylon bristles. These stiff bristles scratch at the delicate scalp covering and, used day after day, irritate and eventually damage the hair and scalp to the extent that balding occurs.

It is not always easy to select a natural bristle that is sturdy enough. They are deceptively firm to the hand, but once in contact with the resistant force of thick hair can become ineffective if you have chosen a too-soft bristle. But this is entirely individual, and you may choose to start with a less firm brush and work up to the sturdier bristles, especially if your hair is heavy in texture. On the other hand, avoid a harsh type of bristle. Use care in selecting your natural bristle brush by choosing one that suits the needs of your hair, is comfortable to use and doesn't scratch the scalp.

Use even movements when you brush. No short, quick strokes, but rather long, even ones, from the scalp to the ends of the hair.

Begin at the nape of the neck and slowly brush all the way around the head until you have returned to the starting point. Brush outward from the hairline, remembering to cover every area of the scalp in order to leave no spot where dust, dandruff, and oil might remain to cause trouble.

It is amazing how relaxing this daily or nightly ritual can become, and how much you will look forward to it. The tension which may also affect the scalp and hair growth, is alleviated by this practice and the entire body becomes relaxed from this slow and calming routine.

Massage

Another help in stimulating hair growth and promoting a healthy scalp can be found in an intensely satisfying self-massage. Some doctors maintain that brushing alone is of little help in aiding hair growth; that the roots cannot be adequately invigorated by surface stimulation. They suggest that only by thorough massage can the hair roots be adequately stimulated.

The method they encourage calls for placing palms flat against the scalp, closing the fingers around the hair at its lowest point, and gently pulling several times before moving to another area.

Certainly, this type of massage is easy enough to practice. After the first twinges, which indicate a lack of tone to the scalp, there is a feeling of pleasure in the massage. If practiced daily, within a short time this toning massage becomes anticipated much the same as an athlete looks forward to a sprint around a field.

Remember to grasp the hair firmly, and to pull gently, just enough to feel the movement below the scalp. If you are losing hair, obviously you would not use this method of stimulation. Nor would this be the correct treatment for any serious scalp disorder. You must first clear up any major distress before practicing this.

Massaging greatly benefits the scalp. But if done too enthusiastically, you can do more harm than good. You don't need a vibrator brush or other special equipment; a good palm and finger massage of the scalp and hair is just as beneficial.

Run your flat, open hand through your hair with your fingers spread apart. Work toward the back, gently rubbing with your palms and pulling gently at the hair with your fingers, always keeping the palm of your hand flat against the scalp as you gather in the strands of hair at their lowest point. Pull gently at an area, slide your palm backward, and continue until all parts of the scalp have been reached.

This stimulating action brings a fresh blood supply to the hair roots and increases their nourishment.

Hair Loss

One of the more shattering experiences in a woman's life is to find excessive quantities of her carefully groomed hair filling her brush, protruding from her comb, or lying on the pillow after she has arisen. Subsequent inspection of her scalp may show thinning hair or even bald spots.

Following the initial shock reaction, a woman usually begins a flurry of shampoo changes and examinations of other hair treatments, including a confrontation with her hairdresser over the possibility that the culprit is her latest dye job or permanent wave.

Hair loss can be due to any one of a number of things, including poor cosmetic practices. Results of the meeting of the first International Symposium on Human Hair confirmed my ideas of what constitutes hair health. Dr. Wilma Bergfeld, a Cleveland, Ohio dermatologist, presented her own findings which proved that excessive shampooing with detergent shampoos is damaging to the hair. She cautioned against indiscriminate use of the multitude of hair products advertised as increasing hair beauty.

At the same meeting, Dr. Algie Brown, a dermatologist from Emory University in Georgia, emphasized the fact that malnutrition can produce loss of natural hair color and curl, and can be the cause of fragility and sparseness of hair (*Atlanta Journal and Constitution,* Nov. 14, 1973).

Neglecting nutrients related to the nervous system in your diet offers an open invitation to poorer hair growth and other body malfunctions. Tension creates muscular contraction which in turn constricts the blood vessels carrying nutrition to the hair shaft. If the nervous tension continues over a lengthy period of time, noticeable hair loss can result from this scalp starvation. And once the hair starts falling out, the usual reaction is an even greater tenseness that generates a vicious and unending cycle.

If you are a harried individual with seemingly endless problems, then your chances of developing thinning hair are greater. The amount of hair you may lose ranges from a coin sized patch of bareness to a huge denuded area.

Calcium can be considered a tranquilizer, and might be just the calming agent that shattered nerves are screaming for. It certainly has proved to be my key to serenity. I used to awaken at odd hours during the night, restless, unable to sleep, and with a curious need to walk. Lack of sufficient calcium had left nerve endings raw and exposed, and created the unrest. Now I pop a few calcium lactate tablets with a cup of warm milk and honey and sleep the night through.

There is really no single way to insure good sturdy hair growth and maintenance. Only a series of combined efforts will correct hair faults. Brushing or massaging will stimulate the healthy scalp, but it is not advisable where there is a fallout problem.

I have received complaints from a multitude of young readers about hair breakage resulting from overuse of curlers. If you prefer a longer hair style, try the pretty simplicity of the straight, flowing style which will eliminate the need of these rollers.

To increase the rate of hair growth, a diet containing all the essentials of good hair health is in order. A sufficient quantity of protein is of primary importance since hair is composed almost entirely of protein. In addition the B vitamins, and vitamins A, C and E are considered important for maximum growth. Minerals including calcium, iron, iodine, potassium, magnesium and copper are vital to maintaining or restoring the hair.

But be patient—according to the medical experts, when hair reaches ten inches in length, any additional growth occurs at one-half the previous rate.

I have found that a B-complex formula taken daily has greatly increased my own hair growth and health. Even though I include in my daily diet the foods specifically containing all the B vitamins, I've noticed an additional spurt of growth that remains consistent as long as I use the potent B-complex formula, heavy on choline and inositol.

Baldness

Baldness among both sexes is on the increase, but men continue to be in the vanguard of this unhappy experience. There have been many theories advanced as to the cause of hair loss, and the theories are as varied as the types of baldness, or alopecia, as it is medically known.

Glandular disturbances and hormonal imbalances, seborrheic dandruff, deficient diet, disease and barbiturates are among the causes cited for hair loss. No one is really sure why more men than women go bald, but one interesting theory states that men have a tighter scalp than do women, with a minimal amount of fatty tissue under the scalp area. This situation can contribute to hair loss, and in turn has been related to the fact that the female head is flatter on top than the male's, and that this tends to reduce scalp tension and permit better blood circulation.

Dr. Irwin Lubowe reports that there is a growing army of women complaining of sudden hair loss, and suggests the possibility that heredity is a factor, since the tendency to bald may be transmitted through genes. Dr. Lubowe says that Dr. E. Sidi, a Parisian dermatologist (plus a great many dermatologists in this country) believes the application of damaging hair cosmetics and injudicious use of reducing tablets contribute to this hair loss problem.

If you have recently noticed that your hair is falling out, check your habits and try to eliminate any factor that is alien to natural living. If you resort to chemical aids to reduce, find a more acceptable way to lose weight. Or if you use sleeping tablets, substitute a cup of warm milk, honey and calcium tablets. And eliminate all hair dressing aids until your problem clears up.

Hair loss after pregnancy is not an uncommon problem, but it is acutely distressing to young mothers. This type of hair loss is generally temporary, and research indicates it is related to a hormonal imbalance as the body seeks to adjust itself. Check your diet to ascertain that you are getting sufficient amounts of essential vitamins and minerals, and don't panic. Dr. Cyril March, Professor of Dermatology at the New York University School of Medicine, says complete regrowth usually occurs with six months.

Hair styles can also be responsible for hair loss. Any style in which the hair is drawn back too tightly will cause extensive damage in its pulling action on the scalp. Hair that is coming out from the scalp rather than breaking off midway indicates damage to the underlying area.

If this is your problem, change your hair style to a looser arrangement. Once this constant pulling on the scalp hair is lessened, your hair should begin to grow back.

A common misconception is that cutting the hair short will make it grow faster. But cutting your hair will not change what is going on beneath your scalp. The best way to improve the rate at which your hair grows is to correct your diet by eliminating excessive animal fats, soft drinks, white flour and white sugar products, and any other non-nutritious foods.

Hair Styles

The person whose hair is thick and fast-growing is blessed, indeed. However, a good hairdresser who can style your hair well is a treasure. If your hair is straight and thick, it can be blunt cut most attractively into whatever style you prefer. This cut is good for fine hair, too.

A layered cut is shaped to the head, and requires more frequent cutting and more attention in setting than a basic blunt cut.

Choosing Your Hair Style

Base your hair style on the shape of your face, your facial features, and the texture of your hair for the most attractive appearance. A hair style can modify a prominent facial feature or emphasize a distinctive shape.

To learn your facial shape, look directly into a mirror and determine which of the following outlines most correctly describes your own: oval, round, square, heart-shaped, wide, diamond-shaped or long.

The person with an oval face can comfortably wear almost any hair style, dependant on facial features. The round face takes a center part well. A square face profits from a rounded out coiffure with feathery curls along the sides. A side part enhances the heart-shaped face, and fullness is added to the lower portion of the face with side curls, or a rounded, chin-length coiffure.

A smooth, close to the face style softens the wide face, while the diamond contoured face responds to bangs and shoulder length hair for flattering width. The long face is attractive with bangs, also, when the hair is pulled softly below the ears and caught in the back.

The wrong hair style is sometimes responsible for infections of the skin. If the skin erupts in those areas where the hair comes in direct contact with it, the hair style should be changed, in addition to taking care of the skin. If your hair is not kept scrupulously clean, germs from your hair may infect your skin. In any event, the hair aggravates the condition. Pull your hair away from your face and be sure you keep both skin and hair clean.

If your hair style requires the use of rollers, be careful in selecting the type you use. The larger the roller, the less damage to the hair, obviously. Never pull your hair tautly onto rollers, for this traction can cause permanent damage. Brush rollers can damage the hair roots if used too frequently and abusively. Never sleep with them in your hair.

Accessories

The convenience of the newly popular blow dryer enables women to shampoo their hair in the morning, dry it in a short while and race off to work. But why do I receive so many letters from users complaining of dry, stick-like hair and dry scalp? Convenience many times exacts a price.

I strongly recommend using the hair dryer strictly as an emergency measure, and taking the extra time to towel dry the hair, replacing the damp towel with a dry one until every strand is dry. The massaging action of towel drying is great stimulation.

Many things that appear helpful prove liabilities in the long run. Though many people believe that their hair is greatly improved by wearing a wig often, my guess is that it just isn't deteriorating as rapidly as before. Stripping, bleaching, dyeing and permanenting, plus using rollers and pin curls, all take their toll of hair. When wearing a wig, perhaps one does not practice these habits as frequently as before and therefore damage is not so rapid.

But I cannot believe that the hair can be covered for a major portion of the day on successive days and not show some damage, either hair loss or a change in the composition, or increased oiliness (which is the complaint of some readers who have worn a wig on successive days).

Wigs are no more natural and desirable than dentures. When really necessary, they are wonderful to have. But it seems foolish to ignore the needs of the body and willfully substitute artificial devices when you can have the real thing.

Chapter 3

Elegant Eyes

When fashions become indeterminate and no single style reigns supreme, eye makeup becomes a focal point. Shaded, shadowed, "mascaraed" eyelids sulk out from under thin or thick eyebrows. Or a wide-eyed innocent look may be promoted, according to the season or magazine you read. And since we all like change, there is a feeling of being adventurous when new styles are adopted and prove wearable. But no matter what style you adopt, it can all be undone by drooping lids or dark semi-circles which are so pronounced even makeup can't conceal the problem.

Moroccan women of the 19th century darkened their eyes by filling a lemon shell with plumbago (a kind of lead ore) and burnt copper and carbonizing it over a charcoal fire. Pounding this into a powder, they added a paste of coral and pulverized pearl, a bat's wing and a bit of perfume. Then they darkened their eyes into dusky allure and no doubt, more than a few women with such cosmetic methods also developed darkening vision to match their eyes.

Spanish women during Lola Montez's heyday were advised to squeeze an orange peel near their eyes in order to brighten them. The oil actually is an irritant and the eyes hastily form tears to rinse away the discomfort. In our own colonial America, in lieu of the luxury orange, women would "flirt" soap suds into their eyes for additional sparkle. I should imagine such practices also created red-velvet eyes from the sting. But if you consider this makeup to be wayout, what about the abundance of paints, glimmers and liners on the market today?

Letters I receive tell me horror stories about applying false eyelashes, individually to each lash, and having the whole shebang fall out in a couple of days, leaving a totally lashless eye. So whether the damage comes in the form of a bat's wing and lead or adhesive to hold an eyelash, I say it is a bad situation.

Care of the eyes is more than a matter of beauty. It has to do with health and comfort, and in order to achieve these tall measures, it is necessary to avoid damaging products and applications and to treat your eyes as the valuable gift they are. And if you are reading this, I assume you are as interested as I am in how to overcome as many problems as possible and accept the results as a reflection of your personal body care habits.

In earlier times, if a girl had poor vision (and less than expressive eyes) she often chose to do without glasses because they were considered unattractive.

One of my favorite stories about the importance of good eyesight comes from my mother, whose own vision remains excellent as she coasts through her seventies. She heard this story from her grandmother, so it's been around a while.

Great grandmother Melissa said one of her nearsighted girlfriends wanted to appeal to a young man coming to call on her, and plotted to overcome any misgivings he might have about her less than perfect vision. Before his arrival, she carefully stuck a large headed white pin into the trunk of a cypress tree at the far edge of the pasture.

As the couple sat on the veranda that afternoon, the weak-visioned romantic said she thought she saw a white headed pin in the cypress tree and suggested they go see. Her friend, properly impressed with her incredible sight, went with her, and on the way she fell over a cow.

An amusing story, for extreme vanity is never an appealing quality. When vision is faulty, corrective measures must be taken in order to extract the fullest enjoyment from life. And probably more people today than ever before are wearing lenses because our life style demands that we use our eyes even during leisure time activities like watching television, viewing movies, and reading.

If you need lenses, wear them. But if you resent them, investigate means of strengthening your eye muscles. There are some excellent books available on the subject.

Lovely Eyes Need Good Light

In contrast to earlier times when men and women remained outdoors in natural rather than artificial light, in this century we begin our day with the lights turned on so we can see the small type in a newspaper. We go on from there to an office or shop where the remainder of the day is spent with more printed matter, or in close work at a machine.

Few offices are well lighted. Either there is glare from poorly placed fixtures or the office furniture is arranged for convenience of space rather than ease in working conditions.

If artificial light is your only source, then do make sure you are using it properly, and if you are suffering from eye strain, insist upon having the lighting system made adequate for good working conditions. Correcting this one area alone can change even your physical appearance, in addition to preventing damage to vision. If poor working habits are continued, in time the ravages will show in your face in the form of lines and wrinkles.

The furrowed brow, the tiny crow's feet, the half squint —all these can indicate poor sight. And for some reason, these are the most difficult to treat wrinkle areas of the entire face. The furrowed brow and crinkled eye skin can be treated best by correcting the cause of poor eyesight and thereby relaxing those areas.

Spend as much time as possible in or near natural light to promote good vision. In fine weather, plan to read out-of-doors. When that is not feasible, roll up the shades, or draw up the blinds, and place your chair by the window. Do the same for sewing or any other close work you have to do.

John Ott, founder and head of the Environmental Health and Light Research Institute in Sarasota, Florida, has shown that good lighting not only helps produce and maintain good eyesight, but that it also advantageously influences other bodily functions.

Crow's Feet

Why would anyone want to imprint unpleasant emotions on her face? Speech is a much simpler means of communication.

It takes fewer muscles to smile than to frown. Try reproducing both of these attitudes on your face and prove to yourself that the lines that form on the face from habitual grimaces are reflections of your inner self. So, be loving and line-less!

Habitual squinting or scowling will embed the radial

lines fanning from the outer corners of the eyes to an unattractive depth if the practice isn't halted and corrected.

Sometimes a simple ironing out procedure with the hands can be helpful in lessening the line depth of crow's feet.

Apply a light cream or oil to the area and open the eyes wide. Firmly press the heels of the palms to each area, allowing the pressure of your palm to expand the area and slightly spread the skin. Maintain this spread for a minute and relax. Repeat two or three more times. Try this daily until you notice improvement.

At the same time, consciously try to eliminate the squinting itself. If your eyes are weak, practice exercises to strengthen the eye muscles. And have your eyes checked to see if you need corrective lenses.

Linda Clark reports on an exercise to reduce crow's feet in her book *Stay Young Longer:*

After oiling or creaming the crow's feet area, close and contract one eye hard. At the same time, lift and contract or tense the entire face on the same side. It looks like a wink plus a smile. Repeat this movement 20 to 30 times per minute for each eye. Eventually increase the practice of this exercise so that you perform it several hundred times a day, or until you accomplish your goal.

Protect Your Eyes

Our sight is one of our most precious possessions, and should be cherished for the gift it is. Yet, daily we commonly strain and tire our eyes by working or reading in poorly lighted areas.

Another hazard is the casual insertion of materials into the eyes. When you use an eye dropper, how clean is it? And what about your mascara brush, has it ever been carefully cleaned? And do you cleanse the area around the openings of squeeze bottles containing eye washes and rinses?

Also, you should know the ingredients in the non-medical eye brighteners, clearers, and the like, which you use. I cannot understand anyone trying a product in the eyes from a drugstore or cosmetic shop, strictly on the advice of a persuasive cosmetician or salesperson. That's irreplaceable sight you're tampering with.

The old-fashioned eye cups that are still widely used as a means of washing the eyes can also be hazardous. These handy little cups are likely bacteria carriers, for generally they are used, rinsed casually, and returned to the medicine cabinet.

Should You Wear Glasses?

Many of us cannot wear contact lenses, yet we don't enjoy wearing glasses, either. There are ways you can improve your vision, and perhaps even eliminate your need for glasses.

While it might not be possible to dispose of your glasses suddenly by switching to foods of high nutritional value, certainly you can increase the strength of your body, and that means your eyes, too, by including those foods that offer the greatest nutrition in your diet.

All of the nutrients which contribute to a healthy body should be considered essential for eye health. But the need for vitamin A is especially stressed in care of the eyes. A deficiency of this vitamin can adversely affect normal eye function specifically by diminishing the ability to see clearly in dim light.

Leafy green and yellow vegetables will help supply vitamin A. The B vitamins are also vital to good sight, and can be easily gotten in brewer's yeast, wheat germ, rice polish and molasses.

Vitamin C should figure heavily in the diet of a person with less than perfect sight. Intake of vitamins D and E, and calcium should be checked and increased if in short supply. Calcium from sunflower seeds is a standby for those of us who have improved our vision by the use of this highly nutritious food.

Dr. Marilyn Rosanes-Berrett believes you can improve your vision and in some instances, dispose of your glasses completely. She maintains that many of 100 million Americans who wear glasses, and the eight million who have contact lenses can benefit from three simple practices. She recommends stimulating the eyes by bathing them in light, swimming the body in a standing position to increase circulation to the eyes, and cupping the hands over the eyes to rest them. Dr. Rosanes-Berrett presents an in-depth discussion on this approach to vision improvement in her book, *Do You Really Need Eyeglasses?* (Hart Publishing, New York).

When an optometrist prescribes glasses, and the prescription is filled, we naturally assume the glasses are right for us. But such is not always the case. A massive study conducted by the Optometric Center of New York, affiliated with the State University of New York, audited correctness of prescriptions and eyeglasses of 8000 persons ranging in age from two years to over 65. Evidence shows 35 percent, or more than one in three pairs of eyeglasses, had incorrectly ground lenses, or incorrect placement of lenses within the frames.

Prescriptions were found to be 15 to 20 percent in error. Another five percent of the patients received prescriptions when they did not require them. Others had their vision distorted by prescribed lenses. Alden N. Hoffner, executive director of the center, says the study was based on patient cards pulled at random from the Medicaid files in New York.

Contact lenses have become extremely popular. In addition to convenience, and for many, improved appearance, contact lenses provide better vision for those persons having undergone cataract surgery. Also, the lenses are frequently prescribed to correct myopia (nearsightedness).

However, not everyone can wear contact lenses. Your ophthalmologist will tell you if you can be fitted for these lenses. A potential wearer must have the proper structure of the eye, eyelid and tissues surrounding the eye. He must also be psychologically able to accept the contact lens as a non-disturbing part of his vision.

Be Cautious With Cosmetics

There have been countless cases of eye makeup contaminated by bacteria and recalled from the market. They have ranged from inexpensive brands to the costliest products from the most prestigious cosmetic firms. Although harmful dyes as ingredients in cosmetics have long been illegal, within the 1970's eye makeup products containing coal tar derivatives which can cause skin cancer have been available. Trying to select a safe eye cosmetic is really like buying a pig in a poke.

I remember hearing my mother say that during the Depression women would strike a sulfur match, allow it to burn for a moment, blow it out, then wet the tip and rub it across the eyebrows to darken them. Sounds old fashioned enough to be safe, but on the other hand, how safe is sulfur? I can't believe it could be any more dangerous than some of today's eye cosmetics that cause irritated, red-rimmed eyes.

One researcher found ten percent of eye cosmetics to be contaminated by bacteria and fungi. Dr. Louis A. Wilson, Associate Professor of Ophthalmology at the Medical College of Georgia, in Augusta, told a seminar sponsored by Research to Prevent Blindness, in February, 1973, that quality control standards permitted some eye cosmetics to reach the consumer in a heavily contaminated state. And while the percentage might be small, he stated those items that were clean on purchase might not remain so, due to questionable preservative practices. He found over 50 percent of used samples to be contaminated.

The principal danger in using eye cosmetics lies in scratching the eye surface with an infected application brush. Severe visual loss can result from these scratches. And never, never use saliva to wet your mascara brush.

Extra Care

Eye beauty, then, is basically eye health. No face can be attractive if it is marred by red-rimmed, streaked or dull eyes. After careful attention is given the eyes, as suggested, there are a few soothing and enhancing extras of eye care one can practice. In Louisiana French we would call them *lagniappe,* a little something extra.

Fight Fatigue

Eye fatigue can be lessened somewhat with calisthenics to strengthen the muscles of the eye. Dr. James Gregg, writing in *Modern Maturity* for April and May, 1974, recommends the following exercises:

Hold your head still and glance quickly to the corners of the room you are in. Glance about for 30 seconds, then close your eyes for ten seconds. Blink your eyes to relieve any tension, and repeat the fixational movements. Close the eyes again and count to ten.

Another quickie eye exercise that might prove helpful is to look steadily at an object on the wall while you roll your head first in one direction and then the other. Next, close your lids and roll your eyes in large circles.

Dr. Gregg feels that any eye movement exercise relieves tension buildup by strengthening eye muscles which, in turn, helps minimize the slowed response of aging eyes.

Borage Eyewash

A borage eyewash can help clear redness stemming from fatigue and, in general, can be used as a gentle bath for the eyes. A mild infusion made from the leaves can strengthen even as it removes strain from eyes stung with cigarette smoke or winter winds.

The demulcent quality of borage insures a soothing cleanser for the eyes when the room-temperature liquid is dropped into the under-lids and the eyes are blinked a few times. Or use compresses dipped into a borage tea and placed on the eyes to relieve inflamed eyelids, or to aid eyes which water excessively. For this tea, use one teaspoon of the dried herb to a cup of boiling water, or a handful of fresh herb to a cup of water.

In earlier days, such herbal brews were used to bathe away puffiness caused by crying. An early beautician suggested it was most unwise for a woman to shed too many tears after the age of 25. It would be detrimental to the beauty of the eyes, she said, for the lachrymal glands are relaxed by weeping and the orbicular tissues (the *orbicularis* is the circular muscle of the eyelid) become emaciated, causing the disfigurement known as drooping eyelids.

Which more or less emphasizes the Biblical quotation: "A merry heart doeth good like a medicine, but a broken spirit drieth the bones."

In any event, borage tea is an unbelievably pleasant way to soothe eyes that have been subjected to excessive weeping, swimming or contaminated air.

Witch Hazel for Tired Eyes

Witch hazel pads placed over the eyes help to reduce temporary fatigue lines if you can patiently lie down for half an hour while they soak away the exhaustion marks. Keep your witch hazel in the refrigerator during the summer for a surprise lift. Douse the pads, squeeze out the excess, lie down, apply, and enjoy! Do not allow the liquid to enter the eyes. The moistened pads will do the work nicely.

Seasonal Irritation

Many people are bothered by smarting, itching eyes during the winter, but have no such problems in summer months. Dr. Spencer Sherman, New York ophthalmologist and consultant to the Society for Visual Care, believes that overheated rooms with their resultant decrease in humidity during the winter months can cause the eyes to smart, burn and itch. This problem is especially annoying to people who wear contact lenses, or those who do not produce enough tears. Cooler temperatures allow the eyes to retain more moisture. So save fuel, and your vision, by turning that thermostat down!

In addition, if you can, get a humidifier to counter the drying effects of the winter heating system. I consider mine to be one of my soundest investments. My apartment, unfortunately, is heated by a gas blower that is really one of the poorest systems I've ever seen. I've lived in many parts of the world, but this modern apartment building settled on a woefully unsatisfactory method of heating. My first winter here saw me frantically trying to keep pace with its damage to my skin. Huge expanses of glass windows require almost continual running of the burner and blower. Not until I purchased a small apartment-size humidifier did my problem disappear. Not only have my skin, hair and eyes benefitted, but my indoor plants have responded with a phenomenal spurt of growth.

Tobacco Smoke Is an Irritant

Irritation of the eyes by tobacco smoke is a major problem for non-smokers, especially those who work with smokers. If you cannot change your colleagues' smoking habits (and there are undoubtedly as many women as men smoking these days), I would suggest changing jobs. Continued eye irritation is damaging and can lead to deterioration of your eyes. Until such time as you make a decision about changing jobs, you might find relief in simple eyewashes. Carry a small bottle to work with you and bathe your eyes once or twice each day.

As part of your defensive action, make it a point to request non-smoking space in restaurants, planes, trains—wherever you go that an indifferent public doesn't consider *your* rights, too. Most airlines offer you a choice of smoking or non-smoking sections. But since the air eventually mingles, why permit smoking at all in public places? On long plane flights I have awakened more than once with a sense of suffocation from restless, sleepless smokers in a long night of travel. This is when a small bottle of eyewash tucked into my handbag becomes worth its weight in gold.

Recent studies made by Smoking Research of San Diego and the U.S. Department of Health, Education and Welfare have established that smoking can be internally damaging to the eyes.

Nicotine constricts blood vessels in the eyes and carbon monoxide decreases the ability of the blood to carry oxygen. The resulting lack of oxygen in the bloodstream limits the eyes' ability to adapt to darkness, and creates the condition known as night blindness.

Visual acuity and color perception are also adversely affected by smoking, but improve when smoking is discontinued.

Goldenseal for Bright Eyes

A solution of goldenseal can freshen, cleanse and ease inflamed eyes. An herbalist shop could supply this useful herb that was first used by American Indians. It brings quick relief to strained and sore eyes.

To prepare the soothing lotion, mix half a teaspoon of the powder into one cup of hot water. Steep and strain the liquid. Dip clean cotton squares into the cooled solution and place over the eyes. Re-dip the squares as they dry, and leave on for 15 minutes.

Camomile flowers brewed in a similar manner will brighten the eyes and ease strain at the same time. Or tea bags of camomile can be moistened with hot water, cooled, and placed directly over the eyes for excellent results.

Your Eyebrows

I know women whose personal grooming is impressive in all areas except the eyebrows. Many women avoid or ignore this area, with the consequent result of an overgrown line of bushy or straggly hair. The brow line should conform to the face—a delicate face can present a leonine appearance if the eyebrows are out of proportion. Similarly, a large woman with heavier features shouldn't affect a pencil-slim eyebrow line.

In removing stray or overgrown eyebrows to achieve today's fashionably thin line, a lot of painful plucking must be done. And each tiny hair pulled out leaves a minute skin opening which allows for the possibility of infection or irritation.

Be sure your hands, tweezers, and skin are clean before you begin the procedure. To cut down on the discomfort, you might apply an ice cube to the area (not near the eye, but on the eyebrow line, or curve), then use your tweezers. Afterward, pat raw honey on the plucked area and leave it on for 30 minutes to an hour, or longer if possible.

I find this greatly reduces the tendency toward redness and irritation.

Honey's attraction for moisture makes it softening for the skin, and at the same time it acts as a natural bactericide.

Too Much

Creating fashionably narrow eyebrows can be an uncomfortable experience for brunettes with a naturally thick brow line. Remember, anything that is actually painful, and alien to your physiognomy, is not really fashionable. You don't have to aim for a thin, arched line of brows. In fact, if your hair is abundant, you are distorting the picture if you appear with delicate, obviously tweezed and arched eyebrows.

Try tweezing out only the wild hairs; that is, those that are both above and below the natural, full eyebrow line. Then, every night and every morning, brush a bandoline, quince or flaxseed type of hairsetting lotion onto the eyebrows, brushing only in the smooth flowing natural line, to hold them in place.

Too Little

The same thing that makes the hair grow also creates fine, full eyebrows and luxuriant eyelashes. Concentrate on protein and check your diet to determine if it has enough of this essential nutrient.

Old remedies for skimpy eyebrows seem to apply today as well as they did yesterday.

Sometimes an application of warm olive oil rubbed gently into the eyebrows nightly will help. This may take weeks to stimulate the proper growth by its lubricating qualities, but it has been lauded for many generations. Always rub the eyebrows in the same direction in order to create a smoother brow line.

Another suggested eyebrow thickener is pure lanolin. For this treatment, dip the fingertips in lanolin and massage into the brows each night. Or try one of the collagen proteins on the market. I've had excellent reports from people using these products.

Luxurious Lashes

In this day of instant eyelashes, perhaps not too many women are eager to grow their own. However, increasing the length of your own lashes can eliminate the daily stabbings that occur from myopic placement of artificial eyelashes.

Castor oil is one means of slowly, but surely, improving the quality of weak or short eyelashes. This coating must be applied nightly for some months before appreciable results will be seen.

Liquid protein solutions also strengthen and encourage eye-lash growth. These, too, would be brushed onto the lashes nightly. But avoid getting too close to the eye itself with these various oils and solutions.

Whatever you do, don't be tempted to cut your lashes in the hope of having them come in more thickly. They won't, and it will take forever for them to return to the length they were before you cut them. Unfortunately, this false notion is still abroad, and is repeated as fact. I learned the hard way. When I was a budding teenager newly conscious of the possibilities of a mass of fluttery eyelashes, my sister Sybil told me if I would cut my lashes halfway off, they would return much thicker. So I did, and they didn't! It took years for my lashes to grow back to their former length. I don't know where Sybil got her information, but I do know she didn't cut hers. It took years for me to forgive her.

A lengthy illness, especially from a virus, may cause eyelashes and brows to fall out. Olive oil would not help in a case where a virus was or is present. In such an instance oil would probably serve only as a lubricant, and it seems that much more is needed here.

Here is one reader's suggestion for stimulating the growth of eyelashes:

"Try breaking open a vitamin D capsule every evening and patting the oil over the lids and into the lashes (you can massage the vitamin into your brows, too, if necessary). I've been doing it for three months and the results are fantastic. No one believes they are for real, especially as I've never been a winner in the hair and lash department. I only wish I could have found this at the age of 20 instead of 50, but it is fun, even now, to have this luxurious growth."

Whether this treatment will work in all cases I cannot

say. Because all needs are highly individual, what works for one may not do so for another. But these little self helps are safe, for we are dealing with natural foods. Do avoid getting the vitamin D oil in the eyes, as it can sting. And do not try to use the tablet form of vitamin D, but rather a natural fish oil source. In capsule form, both A and D are combined.

I've not tried this, but merely pass it on for those who want to try an heroic measure. There is a definite fishy odor to these oils, and it is far from romantic to retire smelling of fish. However, this is better applied at night because of the tendency of the oil to enter the eyes when you are awake.

Beneath Your Eyes

Undereye tissue is quite fragile, and should not be massaged or handled very much. And most facials should not be placed there. Because it has such a scant oil supply, this area readily loses oil to an astringent application, and develops the tight, dry condition so common among women today. When you are applying anything to this area, or even washing your face, do not rub at the delicate tissue; a light patting is all it can endure.

Many women with good complexions who abide by the rules of health develop dark looking "bags" under their eyes, and naturally wonder why. If you find yourself in this situation, first ask yourself, "Am I getting enough sleep?" Our eyes are quick to reflect the state of our bodies, and if you are suffering from fatigue, the unattractive bags will soon appear directly beneath the eyes. Fat pockets can also develop beneath the eyes and become repositories for fluid to produce a swollen effect. In stretching the thin undereye tissue, the area develops a transparency which tends to reveal the darkened material beneath. Generally this is a matter for your plastic surgeon, if the condition bothers you.

Presto Eye Magic

When it is a matter of insufficient sleep or an equally uncomplicated problem, try the fabulous method of steeping two papaya mint or plain papaya tea bags in two cups of boiling water. While the tea is still warm, apply the bags to the area under your eyes. Be sure the tea is only warm, not hot. You will, of course, be lying down in order to hold the tea bags in place. And who knows? You might even fall asleep during the 15 minutes of treatment and all to the good.

Another remedy for bags under the eyes is to use one fresh fig, cut in half and placed directly on the darkened area. Again, for best results and ease of application, apply while lying down. Allow to remain on for 15 minutes or so. Pat in a film of oil after rinsing away the fig juice.

During the summertime, find a fresh-from-the-vine cucumber, grate it and apply instead of the fig.

You should see excellent results from both. You could make this a winter-summer change, using figs whenever they turn up in the market, and fresh, unwaxed cucumbers at other times. Use this remedy as often as you wish until you see results.

A common misconception is that brunettes should expect to have dark circles under their eyes because of their deeper skin tone. Brunettes generally do have a heightened color tone, but this does not necessarily mean dark circles are a natural occurrence. Kidney disturbances will sometimes reflect themselves in a darkening of undereye tissue. Check this out with your doctor. If this is not the case, you might want to try steeping two tea bags until they are only slightly warm, pressing them out a bit and, lying down, placing them over both undereye areas. This will some-times lessen the darkened circles under the eyes. Sufficient sleep is also necessary to eliminate, and avoid, this problem.

Instant Glamor

Here is a fashion model's trick for tightening up sagging undereye tissues:

Rub a very thin coating of unbeaten egg white into the area with your fingertip or a small artist's brush. Then allow the egg white to dry and apply your makeup foundation very carefully over it. Pat in the makeup instead of rubbing it in. The secret of the whole procedure is in the thinness of the egg white application.

This is an excellent practice for those who need a few hours of extra glamor. The lined area directly under the eyes is temporarily smoothed by the drying effect of the egg white. A great trick as long as you realize you will turn back into a pumpkin in no more than three hours! And after removing the egg white, be sure to use an oil or lanolin cream on this area, for egg white is drying to the skin.

Protruding eyes and drooping eyelids often seem to defy treatment. It is believed that one cause of this ab-normal condition is weakened muscles caused by a lack of vitamin E. Adelle Davis suggests large doses of vitamin E taken daily, and describes one patient with severe myositis. After taking 600 units of vitamin E a day for some time, her eyes cleared to a normal condition.

Chapter 4

Have a Super Smile

Dental Care

Though dentures can now be made by some aesthetically-minded dental laboratories to resemble your own lost teeth, in general they remain a glaring advertisement of substitution. And they are never as comfortable or serviceable as your own. Preventive dental care is mandatory to retain your own teeth. This includes a diet that supplies all basic nutrients and is free of processed foods.

A program of thorough cleansing of the teeth and gingiva, or gums, must be employed to remove all debris at least once a day from the oral area. And this requires more than just brushing, for a toothbrush alone is not sufficient to cover all sides of the tooth. As a matter of fact, brushing the teeth does not clean 75 percent of the tooth where plaque forms, nor does a toothbrush reach half of the gingival crevices where dental disease begins, according to Charles T. Peterson, D.D.S., of London, Ontario, Canada (*Pakistan Dental Review,* July/October, 1973).

You cannot afford to be without any nutrients for the overall health of your body. And by getting all vitamins and minerals in the proper amounts, you can be more assured of trouble-free teeth.

Teeth are composed of calcium phosphate, so there must be an adequate supply of this mineral as a repair material. Vitamin D is required for the body to assimilate the calcium. In addition, vitamin A is needed to protect the tooth enamel, while vitamin C prevents tissue breakdown.

Normal cellular development and tooth appearance is affected by a lack of vitamin A, just as a prolonged vitamin C deficiency invites degeneration of the enamel forming cells, which in turn leads to a defective tooth enamel.

Keep Your Teeth Healthy

Dental caries is a deficiency disease, as are most other dental disorders, but hygiene is also of primary importance.

Use a soft toothbrush and brush long enough after each meal —or at least once a day—to remove all food deposits. A toothbrush with rounded edges is preferable to one with straight bristles, for it is less likely to injure the gum line. Vibrate the brush in an effort to remove plaque deposits at the base of the teeth. Cleanse the tongue, too, in order to remove the invisible but damaging deposits of plaque. In addition, use two-by-two-inch squares of sterile gauze to go over each tooth once a day, polishing to remove any adhering matter. Use dental floss each evening to reach the sides of each tooth, and the lower sections just under the gingiva. Add sturdy foods to your diet to help massage the gums.

Warning Signs

Dental troubles like excessive amounts of calculus on the teeth and tender, easily infected gums can be the first steps on the way to periodontal disease. This painful condition will cause the gingiva around the teeth to shrink to the point that the teeth loosen and eventually fall out. Breakdown of the teeth and gingiva doesn't occur overnight, and deficiencies are probably of long standing. An improved cleansing technique coupled with drastically improved diet should help ward off the disease when the first symptoms begin to appear.

Periodontal disease is held responsible for loss of all teeth in 22 million Americans, so it is a very real problem, and one that requires far more than a cursory toothbrush treatment to overcome. In fact, it's that lick-and-a-promise treatment that can start you on the road to losing some irreplaceable friends—your teeth.

Perhaps you can ward off the more serious degrees of dental disease by learning how to recognize dental problems in their early stages.

The grim evidence to persuade you that your teeth and gums are diseased can be found in inflammation of the soft gum tissue, bleeding of the gums, pockets of pus around the roots of the teeth, gum recession and loose teeth.

Deeply stained teeth, and those with deposits near the gum line, plus cavities and poorly aligned teeth are other warning signals. In addition, bad breath coupled with the above can be a symptom of decay or gum deterioration.

For gums that aren't severely irritated, dedicated home care can sometimes prove effective in re-establishing gum integrity.

Careful brushing and flossing can strengthen the area by preventing buildup of additional deposits. And a salt water rinse made from one teaspoon of salt in a glass of very warm water, used with a strong swishing action, can soothe inflamed gums. Repeat the rinse hourly until the gum condition improves (Family Health, *August, 1973*).

For more severe conditions, consult your dentist.

Healthy Gums

Gentle massage of the gums should be practiced in order to strengthen them.

With your finger, rub in and around every tooth daily.

This massage helps to make up for our lack of chewing on fibrous and crusty foods as man did in earlier times. The stimulation received from sturdy foods or the finger massage helps to keep the gums firm. A toothbrush is also helpful if used without pressure.

Dental Care for Children

How can you judge when to start your child on a serious program of dental care? At the risk of sounding facetious, the answer appears to be, before he is born. Protein deficiency during gestation and lactation increases susceptibility to tooth decay, according to investigators Drs. Juan M. Navia and Lewis Menaker at the University of Alabama Institute of Dental Research in Birmingham. Study results suggest protein deficiency and excessive sugar consumption and snacking can result in a higher incidence of tooth decay.

I don't mean to cause panic, but simply to alert you to the fact that dental care, as all health care, doesn't commence at a specific age. It is a responsibility of a mother even before her child is born.

But all is not lost. Develop a good approach to meal preparation and food habits. Instill in your child a liking for wholesome foods and a pleasant attitude, coupled with explanation to your child, as he grows, on the need for dental hygiene. If you start him off on the right path, he can build up a sensible attitude toward dental health that will help him to keep his teeth beautiful for a long, long time.

Cleaning Your Teeth

Certain foods contribute to plaque formation by encouraging the growth of bacteria on the enamel surface and by inducing production of the excess acid that is responsible for cavities.

Using large quantities of raw, crisp vegetables and fresh fruits is of value in good dental care not only for necessary nutrients, but because these foods do not create the plaque that comes from a diet heavy in carbohydrates. Instead, they bring cleansing qualities along with their nutrition.

Commercial toothpastes have come under fire for containing possibly harmful ingredients, yet many people claim that using toothpaste all their lives has never harmed their teeth. According to a Canadian dental surgeon, Charles T. Peterson, D.D.S., one substance used to polish teeth is similar to zircata, a hard glass-like substance that was used for centuries to polish porcelain.

When such a gritty material is employed to whiten the teeth, not only does it abrade the tooth enamel, but it can also damage the protective oral surfaces, cut the gums and cause the tissues to bleed.

Some mouthwashes can remove the protective fatty acids on the teeth and gum surfaces and leave the enamel unprotected. When the gum tissues are cut, and the outside layer of the tooth is destroyed, infection enters into the tooth (*Pakistan Dental Review,* July/October, 1973). Ideally, according to Dr. Peterson, teeth should be cleansed from the foundation, in order to insure a healthy mouth. And dentifrices should not be made with grit, detergents or caustics, but should contain fatty acids and biological compounds which protect and heal the mouth surfaces.

Better Than Toothpaste

There are several mixtures you can prepare at home for brushing your teeth. The old standby, a mixture of soda and salt, remains an effective cleaner. Another formula calls for lightly roasted and ground rosemary leaves, Peruvian bark, mint leaves and powdered charcoal. Some botanic supply houses offer prepared mixes of toothpowders and liquids, as do health food stores.

When I used to visit my grandmother, deep in the Louisiana countryside, I was introduced to the local custom of breaking a twig from the sweetgum tree, peeling off the outer layer an inch or so from the end and chewing on the exposed part until it was soft and pliable. This softened twig became a toothbrush when dipped into a mixture of soda and salt for cleansing the teeth. And one could have a fresh toothbrush for each scouring! I still recall some beautiful teeth among even the oldsters in that region. I'm sure that chewing on the end of the sturdy sweetgum twigs contributed to those lovely teeth.

Apple juice has been suggested as a natural cleanser for the teeth. If you want to try it, just dip your brush into the liquid and brush away.

Pure apple cider vinegar should be avoided as a wash for the teeth—an acid strong enough to remove tartar would probably attack the enamel. Any strong solution can etch the enamel and subsequently expose the underlying areas.

However, Dr. D. C. Jarvis, folk-medicine doctor, recommends a teaspoon of apple cider vinegar diluted in a glass of water to be taken at each meal as an aid in reducing plaque.

The hygienist in your dentist's office can brighten your teeth in a few moments. In between visits, rubbing the teeth with a fresh strawberry is supposed to remove stains. Or rub a lemon peel over the discolored teeth, but be sure to rinse thoroughly.

The Social Scourge

The scores of advertisements that tell us bad breath is a major social offense have caused many people to become over sensitive about their breath. They feel that frequent brushing is not enough protection, even though their digestion and elimination are excellent.

Additional information on this subject comes from Dr. Walter C. Alvarez, who says that while most people have inoffensive breath, many of those who do suffer from chronic halitosis may be reflecting some emotional problem or difficulty. In fact, he believes that this is the commonest cause of bad breath. Other causes can be related to diseased kidneys or damaged liver, or stem from food particles remaining in the teeth and decaying (*Modern Medicine*, February 19, 1973). Bad breath can also come, of course, from decaying teeth. Yet another source of offensive breath is poorly digested food putrefying within the body. When the stomach is lacking in hydrochloric acid, bad breath can be one of many results.

Plaque

Plaque, or calculus, is created by saliva deposited and left on the teeth long enough for the glue-like substance to harden. Saliva is a mixture of glandular secretions, and its composition is influenced by the types of food you eat. Sugar causes a larger amount of plaque to be secreted than do non-sugared foods.

To get rid of plaque, a hygienist or dentist must break up the deposit, removing it from both the exposed and unexposed tooth surfaces. The best way to deal with plaque is to prevent its formation in the first place by careful brushing and cutting down on sugar consumption. Plaque forms, my hygienist told me, every 12 hours. So it becomes necessary to sweep away the saliva adhering to the teeth before it has a chance to seal itself on.

A naval dentist told me, "Move it about! Even if you aren't an enthusiastic tooth brusher, get that deposit off the teeth before it latches on and has to be moved professionally by a hygienist or dentist."

Nobody Needs Cavities

Don't depend on your toothpaste alone to prevent cavities. What you eat has just as much of an effect on your teeth as what you use to clean them.

Dr. Irwin D. Mandel, director of the Division of Preventive Dentistry at Columbia University in New York, says that among people in Southeast Asia, only one tooth in 200 becomes decayed. But the rate is 50 times that high in the United States. He blames the galloping consumption of sugar in this country.

Many dental researchers agree that sugar is a prime factor in creation of cavities—so curb your sweet tooth if you're plagued with this problem.

Do You Really Need Dentures?

Many adults with crooked, unevenly placed teeth are eager to have them removed and replaced with dentures for cosmetic reasons. If the concern is for appearance only, it would be a terrible mistake to have all the teeth removed.

No matter how well-fitted dentures are, they are a poor substitute for your own teeth.

And no matter how bad the condition, complete extraction should be considered only as a last resort. Some dentists maintain that having only a few teeth in the mouth onto which to anchor partial dentures is a far wiser plan than having them all removed, leaving no stable support. Vanity should not be a reason for removing sound teeth. There are too many alternatives; crooked teeth can often be straightened, even for adults. And capping may be costly, but it can be a practical investment if it prevents you from having your teeth removed.

If you must have your teeth removed for health reasons, perhaps you may be able to find a substitute for total extraction. There exists a method of implanting artificial roots into the regular root area to anchor the teeth, thus avoiding the need of false teeth altogether.

The endodontic implant—or stabilizer—has been used for over 20 years in South America, and also for several years in Europe. Endodontic implants have also been performed by a small group of dentists in the United States.

In principle, a rod is inserted through the root canal into nearby bone to act as a root extender, anchoring and supporting the tooth. Check with your local dental society to find out if this procedure is available in your area and if it is practical for you.

Dentures

Some denture-wearers find to their dismay that they develop a long chin and sunken mouth. Properly fitted dentures, of course, are necessary to avoid acquiring an unnatural position of the mouth area while trying to maintain dentures in the most comfortable position. If you have difficulty with your dentures, return to your dentist until they are properly adjusted and you are as free of discomfort as is possible. Dentures, of course, may never be as satisfactory to wear as your own teeth were. They are estimated to be less than half as efficient as natural teeth. But there should be no *major* discomfort in their usage, unless you have some malformation of the jaw or alveolar ridge.

To keep the muscles of the mouth strong, practice the following exercise.

Purse the lips as tautly as possible while forming a small "o" with the lips. Try to force-expand the lips while at the same time resisting making the circle any larger. This play against the muscles in the lip area should strengthen the mouth considerably if practiced several times a day.

Chapter 5

Fabulous Fingernails

Back in 500 B.C., a woman took with her to the grave her own cosmetic kit with instruments for nail care, little different in purpose from today's equipment. Queen Hetepheres, mother of Cheops, was buried with a hand wrought manicure set of seven gold and bronze knives and a metal orange stick with one end rounded and the other sharp, much like the ones sold today.

Probably Chinese women of the ancient ruling class had greater fingernail problems than anyone before or since. With their three- and four-inch fingernails, imagine the time required to replace a broken nail! Consequently, coverings were artistically made of gold, silver or bamboo.

But these long talons with their elegant sheaths seem as useless as a bound foot, and improbable in today's busy world. For most women it is difficult to grow a fingernail to reach beyond the fingertip itself. Many modern fingernail problems stem from the damaging chemical action of detergents and other cleansers. But in addition, there are cosmetic preparations on the market that can do much damage to the unsuspecting user.

So read this chapter to learn what you are putting on your fingernails along with the pretty lacquer that is almost a part of your makeup. But read it also to discover what researchers have turned up about your diet's influence on the fingernails; they are, indeed, a window to the body's internal condition.

What Are Fingernails Made Of?

Fingernails are essentially the same horny tissue as the claws and horns of animals. It is a type of tissue that is nearly pure protein, although its amino acid structure is so unbalanced that it is of no value at all for protein nutrition. Yet even though the nails are composed of what we usually consider low grade protein, it is protein we must feed them. Brewer's yeast is one method of insuring adequate intake of extra protein, in addition to a balanced diet.

Fingernails may one day become as positive a proof of your nutritional state as fingerprints are today of your identity. As found in tests conducted by J. R. K. Robson, formerly with the World Health Organization, measuring fingernail hardness to determine nutritional status is an extremely simple and quite accurate procedure. The test, reported in *Research News,* was devised to accommodate public health officials in areas of the world where technology and manpower are inadequate to employ the standard procedure of measuring body fat, height, weight, and tissue nutrients. By resorting to direct field methods of fingernail evaluation, public health officials would be able to detect malnutrition solely by observing nail texture.

Even marginal malnutrition can be detected by the simple fingernail examination because the range of nail hardness among those receiving an adequate diet is small. In determining why nails harden during malnutrition, researcher Robson found that some of the fingernails tested reveal an absence of zinc, a mineral related to protein metabolism and stunting of growth.

Many of us are impatient with diet as a corrective measure for external complaints. But there is simply no shortcut to the health or attractiveness of any body member. Incredible varieties of nail coverings are sold to harden, lengthen, and "protect" the nails—all out of a bottle, and all as quick ways to nail beauty. But these products do not really overcome your nail problems, nor do they replace corrective dietary practices.

How to Care for Your Nails

Day-to-day care of the nails includes protecting them in every possible way while getting one's chores done. Cotton lined rubber gloves are a must when the hands are going to be immersed in any cleaning solution.

Nothing is better for external care of the nails than a daily buffing. This stimulating action can actually strengthen the nail. And it will also give it a sheen that no amount of lacquer can equal. Find one of the old fashioned buffers, so popular until nail polish came in, in an antique shop and refit chamois skin to it. Or check with department stores. Some have reinstated the chamois covered buffer.

Beauty at Your Fingertips

Nail polishes are not desirable, yet many of us still like to add color to our nails. There are some attractive natural cosmetic preparations on the market that give us our moments of glamor without any harm whatsoever. The cosmetics we try to avoid are those containing harsh and damaging ingredients.

Egyptian women used henna paste to impart an amber shade to their fingernails. They also applied it to their palms and the soles of their feet as a beauty agent. However, we'll concentrate on the fingernails.

Henna Paste

Mix a teaspoon of dried henna powder (purchase it through a botanical supply house in order to obtain the pure plant and not a metallic compound) with enough water to make a medium-thick paste. The Egyptian ladies rubbed the paste into their fingernails and held their hands in the sun for it to dry. Bearing in mind that those unpleasant brown spots on the hands can come from excessive sun exposure, perhaps you might like to allow your nails to dry naturally.

Apply only enough to cover the nails in a thin coating. Rinse off when the powder is completely dry and carefully blot the nails. Buff with light strokes. Remember this won't be a deep color, only an amber tint. But it is safe and attractive.

Keep Your Nails Healthy

Protein is one of the most important nutrients needed for healthy fingernails. For maintenance and repair, a sufficient protein intake is mandatory. The Food and Nutrition Board of the National Research Council recommends 70 grams of protein a day for men and 60 for women. Pregnant women require 85 grams, and 100 grams is deemed necessary for nursing mothers.

However, it is the opinion of some nutritionists that more protein than this is required to keep the body at maximum levels of performance and attractiveness.

Anyone who wants beautiful nails can help them along

with applications of a fingernail food. Feeding fingernails is not so far out as you might imagine. While one's diet to a great degree determines the state of one's nails, as we have seen, there are external practices that can affect them also.

Fingernail Food

For a beneficial external treatment, try mixing equal parts of egg yolk, almond or linseed oil, and raw unheated honey. Massage this mixture into the nails the last thing at night and allow it to remain on overnight, rinsing away in the morning.

Only a thin covering is necessary; the tiny portion that will be absorbed comes more from the massaging action of applying it than from the thickness of the coating. But if you want to insure stain-free bed linens, perhaps you would feel more comfortable wearing gloves (two sizes too large) to bed.

Brewer's yeast can be taken in a variety of ways. Because of its fairly strong taste, you may find it objectionable taken in a glass of water. If this is so, add it to any fruit or vegetable juice. Generally speaking, one tablespoon of dry, powdered, grain-grown brewer's yeast should be mixed into a glass of liquid and taken, in this quantity, three times a day.

You might prefer to work up to the desired three tablespoons a day on a gradual basis. Start with a teaspoon of the yeast to a glass of liquid. Mix it well, until the yeast is completely blended with the liquid.

Adelle Davis suggests, because yeast is high in phosphorus and low in calcium, and because an excess of phosphorus cancels out the calcium, that calcium lactate should be added to yeast before taking it.

She recommends the addition of one-fourth cup of calcium

lactate to one pound of yeast. Mix them thoroughly together before using.

This will insure the fullest utilization of an outstandingly beneficial food.

Make your fingernail therapy a daily practice. After your nails have achieved an impressive growth and sturdiness, continue to take the yeast daily as maintenance.

Some people have found that eating almonds has helped strengthen their fingernails. Many others have heard of the success of this method, but regard such treatment as a fad. I don't consider the pursuit of health a fad. There is certainly nothing extreme in searching out cause and effect, especially as it relates to a feeling of comfort and clears up problems which heretofore defied solution. Eating almonds in an attempt to gain needed nutrients for better nail health seems far wiser (and less faddish) than covering the nails with a lengthener or a layer of plastic in an attempt to solve what is basically a problem of faulty nutrition.

Readers write me of eating five almonds a day over a period of months and finding great improvement in their fingernails. The value of almonds lies in their content of protein, carbohydrate, fat, linoleic acid, thiamine, riboflavin and niacin.

One reader informed me her doctor suggested she eat five almonds a day as a good source of the calcium in which she was deficient to help a different problem, and she subsequently eliminated splitting nails as an extra benefit.

Herbs for the Fingernails

If you're in search of a natural herbal strengthener for fragile nails, add horsetail to your garden. This medicinal plant is favored in England, where herbs used for health and beauty have been more appreciated than here in America. But those who know the value of this weed-cum-herb speak of its high silica content, and perhaps that's the reason for its usefulness as a nail dip.

Herbal Nail Dip

Using dried leaves, make a strong solution of a tablespoon of horsetail to a cup of hot water. Use as a fingerbath as often as possible for ten minutes a day. A daily dunking, if you can manage it, should prove most beneficial in strengthening fragile nails. In addition to the fingerbath, those with unusually soft fingernails might try drinking a mild horsetail tea each day. Since this is a powerful plant, use only half a handful of the herb to one and one-half pints of water. Brew it as a tea and take two dessertspoonfuls morning and night. This would be continued over a period of several weeks or months before improvement would be noticed. Remember, an herbal approach to health and beauty is slow, but reliable.

Soft Nails

You might also try soaking your fingers each night in warm olive oil. This has helped many people. Iodine applied to the nails is another effective strengthener.

Hard, Brittle Nails

Extremely hard nails are no more desirable than nails that are too soft. Studies made of fingernails of malnourished persons show their nails to be markedly harder than those of well nourished people. When the diet is improved, the nails of these same people become proportionately softer. A healthy fingernail is not so soft that it tears and splits, but it is resilient and flexible. Even marginal malnutrition can be detected by fingernail examination. Check your intake of all nutrients and correct your diet, where needed.

For splitting or brittle fingernails, gelatin is an old remedy that has helped some people. Gelatin is made of exactly the same horny tissues of animals that correspond to fingernails in people, and contains (and adds to the bloodstream) large quantities of just the amino acids fingernails need.

The drawback is that gelatin is such unbalanced protein it could easily make you sick if you relied on it alone as a protein source. When adding it to your diet, consider it only as a supplement to feed your fingernails (and hair).

It must be prepared with milk or meat broth to produce a balanced protein. When mixed with another protein source to form a complete protein, one package of gelatin a day can sometimes make nails stronger, more flexible and generally healthier.

Adelle Davis attributes some cases of brittle nails to an iron deficiency. If this is your problem, you will want to increase your iron intake by concentrating on foods like liver, brewer's yeast, blackstrap molasses, apricots and eggs.

Detergents Are Dangerous

We know what harm detergents can do to hands, but not all of us realize that these products are bad for the fingernails, too. Damage from detergents occurs when delicate skin is immersed in a chemical cleanser intended for household chores. I am constantly amazed at people who don't realize that an agent strong enough to strip away grime cannot be expected to leave fragile skin unharmed.

It is not the fault of the cleanser, then, but a matter of an impractical attitude. You can be assured that any cleansing agent that is actually *good* for the skin (or nails or other part of the body) would really be falling down on its job as a cleaner.

The Cardiff Royal Infirmary in Great Britain has confirmed that detergents can cause loss of fingernails.

I have found that women in the more remote areas of the world, who have fewer modern household cleaning preparations, suffer fewer nail problems than those in the more civilized regions.

During a recent visit to the Meta region of Colombia, I made it a point to examine the fingernails of a group of women washing clothes on rocks in a small stream by the jungle's edge. They used bars of strong, yellow soap they had purchased in the same vilage shop where I bought chili peppers and yucca root.

The women's fingernails were strong, pliable, beautifully oval and sturdy. Eight hours north of San Martin, across the Andes by horseback and bus, I found another group of young and middle aged women scrubbing on the banks of the Magdalena River. Though their hands were coarsened by the cold water and harsh soap, these women, too, had strong, well shaped fingernails. None of them seemed to suffer the unduly soft or brittle fingernails that assail their North American sisters who have automatic washers, foaming bleaches, acrid detergents, and other miracle cleansers.

Nails That Split

Nails that split across from one side to the other are usually weakened by a nutritional deficiency.

The best solution is to check your diet to discover what essen-

tials for good hair and nail growth are missing. Try also a weekly application of white iodine over and under unpolished nails. Then keep them away from your mouth.

Another excellent strengthener is apple cider vinegar. Dip your fingernails into the pure vinegar nightly, just before you retire, for a couple of weeks and see if this helps.

Ridged Nails

A most frustrating problem is fingernails that become ridged and paper thin and seem to grow in layers. Often, bits of the nails break off and leave rough edges.

An anemic condition can cause this lengthwise ridging of the nails. Check with your doctor if you are afflicted with this problem. You may want to increase your natural iron intake with such foods as brewer's yeast, blackstrap molasses, wheat germ, liver, egg yolks and whole grain cereals. A vitamin A deficiency can also cause nails to tissue off, so plan to increase your intake of this vital nutrient, also. I would suggest you use an emery board, rather than a nail file, to remove rough nail edges. An emery board is less damaging to fragile nails.

White Spots

Small, white spots which appear on the fingernails from time to time are believed by some to be caused by bruising the nails. Actually, the cause of these spots, which have long been a cosmetic concern to women, is rooted more deeply within the body than the nail covering. Carl C. Pfeiffer, M.D., in a report to the *Journal of the American Medical Association,* April 8, 1974, points out the fact that though white spots frequently appear on the nails of the index and the little finger of the dominant hand, and can be caused by a blow to that area, more important factors are involved. For those who have such marks will also have similar white spots on the toenails. Dr. Pfeiffer links the occurrence to a zinc and pyridoxine deficiency.

Dr. Pfeiffer states the minimum daily requirement of zinc is 15 milligrams, but diet analysis shows only 11 milligrams as the maximum intake for the average person. And this amount may not be totally absorbed because of the copper present in drinking water or vitamin and mineral supplements.

Fungus Infections

Fungus infections around the nails are extremely distressing, particularly because they tend to recur despite medication. Sufferers describe medical treatments they receive with varying results, most of them disheartening.

Nutritionist Adelle Davis reported that oral antibiotics, by destroying valuable intestinal bacteria, can cause fungus infections to develop not only internally, but also in the fingers and under the nails. Daily intake of yogurt or acidophilus milk could help restore the intestinal flora. Fungus infections can also occur where a vitamin B deficiency exists.

False Fingernails

Plastic fingernails have become quite popular among women whose own nails don't grow well, especially women whose careers dictate that their hands and nails always look impeccable.

In her book on damaging cosmetics available to the public, *Cosmetics, the Great American Skin Game* (Ballantine Books), Toni Stabile reveals some injuries from fingernail products. One manufacturer of plastic nail covers originally denied any harmful effects from the product, even though the FDA received nearly 1,000 complaints from women who had suffered injuries from applying false nails.

Some users found their nails becoming sore, discolored, and brittle, with continuing deterioration. Loosened nails falling away from their beds, black spots, ridging, and infections were some of the damages incurred. Other injuries included flaking and an upward curving of the nails. If you use plastic nails, you must follow instructions explicitly and not wear them beyond the time indicated as safe.

Hardeners

Brush-on nail hardeners may seem a convenient way to treat weak nails. But they can cause quite unexpected effects.

According to Toni Stabile, fingernails have been a recurrent subject of mass injury from cosmetics applied to them. In cases of injury related to nail hardeners, the products contained formaldehyde, a strong sensitizer. It would be far wiser to work from within to boost nail strength than to depend on powerful solutions and lacquers to supply the qualities you can get from an improved diet.

Lengtheners

Some women have success with fingernail lengtheners, but many others exhibit severe allergic reactions to these solutions. Recently, distribution of 450,000 bottles of fingernail lengthener was halted by a federal judge. A chemical in the product caused users to faint, and their nails developed a fungus infection or dropped off after the product was used. This was the first time an injunction against a cosmetic manufacturer had ever been issued on a nationwide scale, according to Assistant U.S. Attorney Frederick Branding (*Medical World News,* August 9, 1974).

Polish

I would never recommend a commercial fingernail polish as totally safe for everyone. As I have stated before, my research shows that many of these nail cosmetics are damaging. Reactions to such applications are many and varied. Dr. Alexander Fisher, Clinical Professor of Dermatology at the New York University Bellevue Hospital Center Skin and Cancer Unit stated in *Medical World News,* July 9, 1974, that he had treated 15 people in recent years who used nail preparations causing sensitized reactions from methyl methacylate monomer, a chemical employed as a polish hardener. Even though the monomer is applied with a protective cover surrounding the nail, residual monomer can reach the skin, according to an FDA report.

While I do not say that no one should wear fingernail polish, and certainly many people experience no difficulty whatsoever, I could not recommend any particular one to be used with guaranteed safety.

Removers

Try to avoid frequent use of the polish removers, for they contain acetone, a strong solvent. And be sure to wash your nails thoroughly after use of a remover. This should help minimize the danger.

Dirty Nails

Almost universally, gardeners complain of dirt under the nails, even when gardening gloves are worn.

Try digging your nails into a piece of suet, pushing cold cream under the nails, or scraping your nails across a bar of softened soap before you go out to the garden.

This will act as a barrier and prevent minerals in the soil from staining the under portion of your nails.

Cuticles

There is one cardinal rule that any of us with creeping cuticles must never forget: *never cut the cuticle.* You will end up with a ragged cuticle that can then become infected, and in any event, will be sore and unattractive. Cuticle scissors seem to be more of an instrument of torture than a cosmetic aid, and are to be avoided at all cost, except for clipping hangnails, if you have that problem. Frequent use of cuticle scissors results in hangnails and bleeding cuticle skin more often than a smooth, oval base for the fingernail.

Use a nail brush to wash the nails and cleanse the surrounding skin. Then gently push back at the cuticle with the corner of a towel or an orange stick. Do this each time you wash your hands.

Chapter 6

The Body Beautiful (Upper)

Pride in the body should be instilled in children so that later years won't find them, as adults, bewildered by the results of years of neglect. A person who really cares for herself will pay at least as much attention to her body's needs as she does to her job, house, garden or her favorite hobby. Learn to like yourself enough to be concerned about your body and to spend time caring for it.

It is said that a woman's age shows most clearly in her elbows and hands. But any area of the upper body can be cruelly revealing if you've ignored its needs.

What can you do with a calico neck, aging elbows, a thickened waist, and full blown hips? And what can you do with neglected and unattractive hands except sit on them to hide them? In Austria women used to sleep with their hands tied above their heads. This caused the blood to drain downward, supposedly making the veins smaller, and the hands therefore more attractive.

Today we know far more comfortable ways of caring for the body. How much better than the painful waist cinchers of our great grandmothers' time are a few waist whittling exercises!

Where Are You Showing Your Age?

The underarm from the shoulder past the elbow speaks quickly of neglect, lack of exercise and casual living. The neck, too, will glaringly reveal the fact that we've lost weight, had an impressive number of birthdays, or spent too much time in the sun.

Usually, when the neck begins to crepe up and accordion-like folds develop, our first response is to buy some cosmetic and lather on a generous amount of the coverup that promises miracles. Then we powder over it and hope we can get by.

Perhaps we can coast on the effects of the cosmetics for a while. But the piper must be paid, and the day comes when the deepening crevices stubbornly refuse to be camouflaged any longer. Then we resort to our last trick. We tie scarves in clever ways to appear a casual accompaniment to our dress. We'll select a pin to give an extra fillip to the scarf, and then we sally forth, confident that we've whipped this thing at last.

But we can't go to bed with a scarf. Or we could, but it's not very chic. And besides, we'd probably get strangled by it. So we wish there were another way. And there is; a much more effective way than either of the two futile coverups.

There are exercises for this trouble spot just as there are exercises for overpadded hips, enlarged abdominal areas, and for the face and all other parts of the body. There is also a helpful astringent cream that will soften and nourish a weathered neck.

Under the Chin

After losing a substantial amount of weight, you may find the skin directly beneath your chin slightly flabby.

A regimen of exercise should always accompany a diet program. Otherwise, as subcutaneous fat is lost beneath the skin, you will find the stretched skin has lost its support.

For toning and tightening the underchin, try the turtle exercise. Daily practice will firm both skin and muscle at the base of the chin and throat.

Push your neck out as far as it will go without following with your shoulders. Now slowly pull the chin inward toward the throat as far as you can. Relax and repeat several times. If you touch this area with your fingers while performing the exercise, you will feel the powerful movement of muscles under the skin. Do this in a slow, easy manner to avoid constricted muscles, and a sore neck.

Underthroat Toner

In addition to the exercise, a stimulating underthroat cream should be of help.

Beat together one egg white, one teaspoon of mint extract, one teaspoon of liquid camphor, one teaspoon of honey and one tablespoon of milk. Pat the mixture onto the throat area and allow it to dry. Rinse away with cool water, blot dry, and apply a thin film of oil, carefully blotting away the excess.

Use only for the throat area and not the face.

You Don't Need a Stiff Neck

If you've wondered why your neck shows definite signs of age that the rest of your body doesn't display, try this simple test.

First, find yourself a comfortable sitting position, either on the floor or in a straight chair. Hold your back straight, spine upright. Allow your head to fall forward limply, and rotate it a few times.

Do you hear a grinding, gritty noise, as though gravel had somehow gotten into your body?

This sound springs from lack of use, and though we associate it with age, many young people experience this crackling sound when they first begin to exercise the neck area. Fortunately, it can be remedied. The sound is actually the accumulation of calcium deposits which can be eventually exercised away.

Although one chiropractor I know says this is a misalignment of the neck position, which can also be corrected, I have known the condition to be improved simply with daily neck exercises. Lack of use of the neck muscles can contribute to this crackling sound, and the condition can be found in both young and old.

One especially beneficial yoga exercise teaches you how to create a smoothly turning head on formerly stiff neck muscles. By loosening this rigid condition, the rotating neck movement will also eliminate tensions which tend to accumulate in this area. And this muscle strengthening practice will bring you the relaxation so sorely missing at the end of a day that has been spent hunched over a desk, or that has seen you deeply absorbed in a heavy schedule that immobilized your body for long, tiring hours.

Sit in a comfortable position and begin to breathe deeply, in and out. Hold the shoulders back and roll the head slowly backward toward the spine. Then, just as slowly, roll the head forward until the chin rests as close as possible to the chest. Return the head to an upright position and then move it slowly toward the right shoulder. Repeat the movement toward the left shoulder.

Continue the deep breathing and slowly rotate the neck to the right, and on around in a circle as though your neck were on a ball bearing. Keep the shoulders straight without moving them.

Only the head and neck join in this movement. Relax, and repeat this movement by rotating the head to the left.

Calico Neck

Due to uneven pigmentation of the skin, the neck may develop patches of discoloration from exposure to the summer sun. The blotches generally fade during the winter, but they are a real cosmetic nuisance in warm weather.

Yogurt is very helpful in fading these unattractive discolorations. But it has to be administered daily until results are noticed. Once or twice won't help to remove what has been termed a "calico neck."

Apply the yogurt to a freshly cleansed neck and throat, after having removed any traces of cleansing cream or makeup with a good scrubbing followed by an astringent lotion. Pat in the yogurt and allow it to remain at least 30 minutes before removing. Overnight applications are even better, rinsing it away in the morning.

Buttermilk will have the same effect. Or, if buttermilk is not available, squeeze lemon juice into sweet milk until it curdles, then drop in the lemon rind to soak for 10 to 15 minutes. Apply the thickened milk to the discoloration and allow it to dry. If there is any stinging of the skin after the milk is rinsed away, rub in a bit of salad oil to soothe it.

One last tidbit on the neck area. In our grandmothers' time, in order to tone their skin, women would gather a bowl of snow and rub it vigorously on the face and neck. Then they would use a turkish towel to dry it with a vigor that brought a glow.

We can produce the same effect with an ice cube wrapped in a face cloth. Only don't rub vigorously so much as pat at the face with the wrapped up ice cube.

This makes a refreshing treat for a summer afternoon.

You're as Old as Your Back

In beginning a self improvement program to ward off the unpleasantness of premature aging, attention should be given to the condition of the back and its posture, for age is revealed here as clearly as it is in the face.

When the spine ceases to be limber, physical movement slows and stiffness and rigidity set in. Poor posture then becomes habitual, and can end in rounded shoulders, thickened waistline, and other undesirable and uncomfortable conditions.

When the spinal column loses its flexibility, surplus flesh begins to accumulate around the shoulders; rolls of unattractive flesh spread around confining undergarments, and the overblown, middle-aged look intensifies, no matter how youthful and well preserved the face.

In addition, when muscles slacken and grow weak from lack of use, skin folds begin to appear. In order to avoid this flabby look, preventive exercises should begin early in life. However, if you have neglected your body and find yourself in the middle years with damage already evident, there is still a chance to reclaim your body and grow younger in appearance and in feeling.

If you think of your vertebrae as the main support of your entire body, you will usually remember to stand tall and to maintain the posture that eliminates rounded shoulders. In order to know what shape your spine is in now, try the back-check test.

Stand upright with your back pressed against the wall. Place your feet together with the knees slightly bent to accommodate this position. Slowly start pressing your spine to the wall, beginning at the lowest part and gradually working up the full length of your spine. Your knees will begin to straighten as your back presses toward the wall.

It is unlikely that you will be able to press the entire length of your back against the wall with your first efforts. But continued practice will eventually make it easy, and will strengthen your spine to the point that the straightened position will help to eliminate the ungainly swayback look brought on by poor posture. In addition, the abdomen will be pulled up and abdominal muscles will receive a toning that will increase their elasticity and help to eliminate bulges there.

Eating the right foods can go far toward keeping the body young, but exercise is also a vital factor in the fight against growing old. A youthful spine will do a great deal for an anti-age program. Developing a rigid back encourages various discomforts and ailments. Real health and comfort are assured only when the spine is kept supple.

Sit on the floor and imagine your body to be a ball. Round your back by dropping your head to your knees and wrapping your arms around them. Give yourself a gentle rocking motion, gain momentum and roll backward, keeping the head tucked into the knees. As you roll backward onto the floor, give yourself a push forward by rolling the body forward several times.

If you roll sideways the first few times, don't give up. Gather yourself together and start over. Remember to keep your head tucked downward or you will fall backward and be unable to roll.

Continued practice will help create flexibility in the stiffened vertebrae, and bring on a youthfulness of movement and a toning of the entire body. In addition, body tenseness that hunches shoulders and carves lines in the face will begin to disappear. Flexing the entire vertebral length induces relaxation of the neck muscles.

I have seen both men and women regain control over formerly unwieldy bodies just by practicing this comforting exercise. I also recall an extremely overweight woman who became so frustrated over being unable to gather her body into a ball that she dieted until she lost enough weight so that she could rock backward and forward without falling sideways. The combination of diet and exercise paid off; eventually she developed a slender, more youthful body.

Posture Is Important

Poor posture is not only unattractive, it is also not good for the body. When the spine is allowed to slump and the shoulders are hunched over, the body's internal organs are pushed into a smaller amount of space than is normal and desirable for proper functioning.

Aside from beneficial exercises to help correct poor posture, it is a good idea to learn to carry your head in a manner that will pull at slumped shoulders and help you to keep them erect at all times. If you put the following practice into effect, you will improve the neck area, including the underchin, in addition to your carriage.

From the moment you arise in the morning, hold your head as though there is a string in the middle of your skull holding it up. Think of your head being kept perfectly balanced by the imaginary cord. This will help to align your spine in its correct position.

The person with a swayback can run into all sorts of difficulties. First of all, you may never seem to fit into clothing the way you should. The dip in your back makes you look caricatured instead of designed, and it is difficult to maintain a flat stomach.

The condition of swayback is usually brought on by an imbalance in posture. Those with this extreme stance—which throws the shoulders backward and the stomach forward—generally walk on the heels rather than the balls of the feet, as they should. Such incorrect placement of weight onto the heels throws the body off balance and to compensate for this manner of tipping backward, the stomach is thrust forward.

This abnormal hollowing of the back can be very effectively dealt with through a couple of exercises, practiced daily.

To begin correcting this poor posture, daily barefoot practice is necessary to restore normal balance to the body.

During every practice session, stand as straight as possible. Now roll your weight from your heels onto the balls of your feet. You should immediately feel a shifting of weight and a straightening of the entire body. If done correctly, your body will now be in alignment.

Practice this rolling forward at different times during the day until the practice becomes routine habit.

To strengthen the weak back muscles that have either resulted from or helped create this condition in the first place, try this exercise:

Lying comfortably flat on the floor in loose clothing, raise the right knee toward the body and bring it back as close to the chest as possible, simultaneously flinging both of your arms behind your head to touch the floor. Repeat the exercise using the left leg and both arms.

The back stretch is also excellent for strengthening the swayback. However, care must be taken not to impose a strain on the weakened area. Do not press forward in this position. Go only as far as you comfortably can. Daily exercise will gradually limber the spine to the point where you can manage the complete movement without strain.

Sit comfortably on the floor, with your legs straight before you and your spine held erect. Lift your arms straight in front of you, in a line with your legs, and gently stretch as far as your arms will let you. Keep your knees straight on the floor. The ultimate goal of the exercise is to grasp your feet in your hands. But you are not to press for this position. Instead, practice the movement daily, and bit by bit you will become aware of your spine stretching in a way that has brought no discomfort.

Above all, do not rock forward in an attempt to reach your feet with your hands. Go only as far as you can in one smooth movement without force of any kind.

The Upper Back

Today's clinging fashions draw attention to almost all of the problem areas of the body. A major area of concern is the roll of fat which many women develop over their upper back, which can give a matronly appearance to an otherwise well proportioned figure.

The surplus flesh which lies just beneath the shoulders is an indication of too little exercise of this part of the body. It is not an easily accessible area, but the following exercise will help to firm the padded back, and at the same time, will give a stimulating pull to lazy shoulders and aid in better posture.

Bend your knees to the floor and place your hands down flat. Drop your elbows to the floor in front of your knees and move the knees back one foot in space. Breathe deeply in and out and raise your legs up straight with unbent knees while keeping your feet, elbows, and hands on the floor below you. All body weight will be on the feet and arms. Slowly raise your head as high as possible. Bend the knees slowly and return them to the floor. Relax and repeat. It is the final upward thrust of the head that pulls on the back shoulder area to invigorate and exercise those muscles.

The Bust

An ample bosom is unfortunately often considered an essential aspect of feminine beauty. There are no gimmicks and no exercises that will make small breasts grow larger, in spite of multi-million dollar advertising to the contrary. But promoters still offer various gadgets, creams and exercisers to a hopeful public. You *can* firm the breast area with daily exercise of the pectoral muscles of the chest area. By increasing the tone of these supportive muscles, you can improve the appearance of your breasts; they will be firmer and appear larger.

An excellent and easily practiced exercise is to sit cross-legged on the floor. Sitting upright, bring your arms around to the back. Holding the palms together toward the base of the spine, slowly bring them up as high as possible, traveling up the spine. Keep your back straight. This may be difficult in the beginning, but continued practice will greatly strengthen and tone the breast area.

Another breast-firmer requires sitting or standing upright and pressing the right fist against the left palm as forcefully as possible. Alternate between the right and left fist several times. Repeat at intervals during the day, but start slowly and gradually increase the number of movements.

The Waist

Now that girdles and corsets have fallen out of favor with the fashion world, women no longer rely on these devices to create an artificial figure. One of the great problems that appears in the freedom of today's fashions is a disproportionately heavy waist. Fortunately, there are many effective exercises to whittle down the waist.

When we want to reduce a block of wood we hold it to a lathe and allow the friction of movement to pare it down to the right size. The same holds true of the waist, only we use the body itself as the reducing machine.

Stand upright and clasp your hands lightly over your head. The head will be centered between the arms. Breathe deeply in and out and swing slowly to the right, keeping the feet in place as your arms and upper torso complete a long, slow swing around the front part of your body. Continue on around to your left until you have described a full circle. Repeat the circle in the other direction. Gradually increase the number of performances until you are practicing this movement several times each day.

Holding the Line

Many readers ask me why their girth expands the minute they turn 40. Almost without exception, women tell me, as of the fortieth birthday, a ballooning of the abdominal area commences and their figures begin to deteriorate. The truth of the matter is that neglected bodies tolerate years of underactivity and overeating, and finally, with no elasticity left in overstretched tissues and with indolence and sensuous dining taking priority over pride of appearance, the body rebels and presents such a person with the results of months or years of indifference to its needs.

The abdomen is one of the most difficult areas to keep firm and flat. When overeating continues, with the subsequent daily stretching of the stomach wall, this part of the body can stubbornly resist rehabilitation. But persistence *will* win.

Don't be discouraged because your abdomen remains large after you have reduced your caloric intake. Dieting alone will not produce the flat tummy that is so attractive in profile. You must consider proper exercises along with your careful selection of food. And though you may have "cut down" on foods that cause overweight, perhaps you have not cut down enough. Why not simply "cut out" all those foods that are not contributing to your overall health, but merely adding extra pounds to your frame. These demons include snacks of potato chips, soda shop specialities, pies, cakes, pretzels, pizzas, hot dogs, hamburgers—the list goes on and on.

In their place use as many natural foods as possible, such as fresh fruits and raw vegetables, sunflower seeds, raisins, apricots, and dates. In addition, try adding an active sport to your day, such as swimming, bicycling, or hiking.

An efficient yoga exercise for trimming a flabby abdomen is the alternate leg raise. This disciplined movement works at the slackened flesh of the entire abdominal area to restore muscle tone.

Lie flat on the floor with your hands alongside your body. Breathe deeply in and out and raise one leg as high as you comfortably can, aiming at a 90 degree angle, perpendicular to your body. Keep the knees straight, both the one on the floor and the raised one. Exhale as you slowly lower the leg. Repeat the exercise with the right leg and then raise both legs at one time and slowly lower them to the floor before repeating. Build up to doing this several times for each position. But do not exercise more than is comfortable.

A variation is to lie on the floor as for the alternate leg raise, but instead of lifting the legs overhead, raise them only two feet off the floor and very slowly lower them. Work up to ten of these twice a day.

Contrary to popular opinion, sit-ups are not among the best abdominal exercises for the average person. Dr. George Coder of Lancaster, Pennsylvania, informed me that much back damage results from the oft-practiced sit-ups. "It isn't so much the strain directly on back muscles that is so damaging," he said. "Rather, it is the fact that in cupping the hands around the neck, permitting the ascent and descent of the torso, the hands can push the neck out of alignment and the pain is felt in the spine." He recommends the exercise I have described to replace sit-ups.

Regaining Your Figure After Pregnancy

After the great stretching of abdominal muscles during pregnancy, dedicated effort is required to regain one's former measurements. But there is one excellent exercise almost anyone can perform to regain elasticity of muscles and toning of the abdominal flesh.

Kneel on the floor with the hands and knees flat. Take a deep breath and drop the head as close to the chest as is comfortably possible. Exhale and suck the stomach in toward the spine, and hold your breath for some moments before relaxing.

Another terrific stomach tightener requires that you pull the stomach backward toward the spine as far as possible. Consciously lift the stomach upward, outward, and then roll it downward, as though the entire area were a ball. Repeat several times, performing very slowly.

Stretch Marks

Stretch marks from pregnancy come more easily to taut, dry skin. Try massaging cocoa butter into the abdominal area at least twice a day until your child is born. Cocoa butter is not really greasy if rubbed thoroughly into the skin, and it will create greater resiliency that can help prevent the forced expansion marks. You should apply the cocoa butter to the buttocks, too, for stretch marks can occur here in addition to the abdominal area. They can also appear on the breasts.

Some scoff at this procedure and call it an old wives' treatment. But who is better qualified to offer information on a problem the medical world hasn't yet solved? The clincher for me was a friend who said she faithfully massaged cocoa butter into her abdomen for all the months she was expecting her child. Not *one* stretch mark appeared, she said, even though she had gained an additional 20 pounds.

The Hips

One of the great demons of women in the business world is a tendency to accumulate excess flesh over the hips from sitting at a desk all day. If corrective measures are not taken, these fatty deposits may grow quite large and unattractive. Once acquired, "saddlebag deposits" can defy all attempts to remove them. Some doctors in extreme cases perform surgery, known as *lipodystrophia,* on this area, but generally it is discouraged because large scars remain as the aftermath.

You might try a side leg lift exercise and keep at it with dedication for some months to see if this helps.

Lie on your side, head comfortably propped on your palm which is, in turn, supported by your bent elbow. Slowly swing your left leg upward as high as it will go, before dropping it down again. Then turn on your left side and repeat the procedure. Continue alternating right side, left side several times for each side. The frequent change from right to left creates additional toning as you roll over on your buttocks.

This exercise requires a long time in practice before any improvement is noticeable, for the condition seems difficult to clear up.

You Can Have Lovely Arms

For the man who said he could tell a woman's age by her elbows and hands, though it may be disloyal to tell him, he could also regard the upper arm as a pretty accurate indicator of age. Women don't seem to observe this part of their body, or else they are indifferent to its ability to sag and loosen.

This is not an easy part of the body to exercise. Yet anyone who uses his or her arms throughout the day usually has firm flesh in the underarms. But how many of us *do* put our arms to use in a working manner? While our legs carry us upstairs and down, indoors and out, our arms are usually suspended by our sides.

A yoga exercise called The Bow not only helps to tone the arms, but does a great deal for other body areas as well. We'll concentrate on the upper arm for the moment, and the extra benefits will come as a pleasant surprise.

Lie flat on the floor, face down, and reach behind you with both hands to grasp your ankles. Lift your head upward from the floor and holding your arms straight, pull upward with your arms raising the knees in order to form a bow. Hold the position for a few moments, relax, and repeat.

Now try the following procedure.

Stand with your arms held directly before you, palms facing downward. Bend your elbows down as you hold your palms upward directly above your shoulders. Very slowly raise both palms directly overhead at the same time as though you were lifting a heavy box. Once the arms are stretched directly upward, support the imaginary weight for a full minute before slowly lowering the box downward. Maintain the exertion in the underarm area rather than the shoulders alone. Start with one complete movement each day and gradually increase the number.

180

Elbows

Hard, crusty elbows may not seem to respond to applications of creams or oils. But don't despair! First, check your diet to determine if you're receiving sufficient vitamin A. Then, why not combine all the beneficial things you've tried separately, and come up with a super cream that really works!

Super Elbow Cream

Blend together a few drops each of salad oil, lemon juice and honey. Rub into the elbows several times a day, and in a week's time your problem should be greatly diminished.

How to Keep Your Hands Young

I receive countless pleas for help from women whose hands are chapped and red, and even painful. The first step in solving this kind of problem is to examine your personal routine; whether your hands are in water a great deal, as a beautician or homemaker, or whether you are an avid outdoorswoman involved in winter sports. For the first two situations, wearing rubber gloves whenever you put your hands in water will do wonders. For the outdoor buff, rubbing in a good hand cream before going outdoors, plus wearing gloves, would offer protection. In order to overcome the chapped hands look, you might like to try the following procedure.

Each night before going to bed, soak your hands in a bowl of whole milk for at least five minutes. Blot very lightly and rub a mixture of three parts of lanolin melted with one part of nut oil (sesame seed, apricot, etc.) into the hands, extending past the wrist. Then pull on a pair of loose kid gloves and wear them all night. Try this for one month, and you should see impressive improvement in your hands.

One is always searching for a heavier cream, a better emollient, or an oilier concoction with which to coat dry hands. But the problem is often due to soap which removes the natural acid mantle from the skin and replaces it with an alkaline coating which dries the skin and produces the parchment-like texture familiar to so many of us.

Even if you use soap, you can remove the harmful alkaline effects by keeping a small container of apple cider vinegar by the washbasin. Sprinkle a few drops into your hands, add water and proceed to rub this solution over your hands.

Many of us can remember, if we think hard, our grandmothers wearing gloves to bed once a week. It may have seemed silly, but remember how lovely their hands were? Our grandmothers were following a practice that is centuries old. Cosmetic gloves have long been used by women who are willing to go that extra mile in beauty care. And it pays off. Want to duplicate their success? Try the following antique formula for beautiful hands.

Grandmother's Hand Cream

Beat one teaspoon of rice flour into two egg yolks until you have a smooth paste. Blend in four teaspoons of sweet almond oil and one ounce of rose water, orange flower water, or elderflower water. (Plain mineral water will suffice if you can't obtain the others.) Beat in very slowly one-half teaspoon of tincture of benzoin, drop by drop. Pat this into your hands before retiring, and have ready a pair of old white kid gloves, several sizes too large. Leave on all night and rinse the hands, without using soap, in the morning.

Clean Your Hands Without Soap

Soap is convenient and it cleanses the hands. That is why we use it. But there are other ways to wash the hands, and eliminate the drying, harsh action of most soap.

Keep a small bowl of bran near your wash basin. Moisten the hands, dip into the bran and rub it thoroughly over your hands to cleanse them. The bran provides friction for cleanliness, and has a softening effect at the same time. Rinse away and feel the smoothness.

The milder cleansers are not effective on hands heavily stained with more than the usual accumulation of grime.

To remove some lighter stains from the hands, rub them with a piece of grapefruit or lemon peel. If the stains are embedded, you might try powdered pumice stone and lemon juice. After such a strong cleansing, though, it is necessary to apply a rich, lanolated cream.

An excellent cleanser for sensitive hands is a mixture of corn-meal and lemon juice. Finely ground Indian meal would be the best, as ordinary cornmeal seems a bit too coarse. Stains coming from tar, or tar products are easily dealt with by rubbing them on the outside of a fresh orange whose skin has been scratched to permit the oils to seep out. For oil stains, try rubbing the hands with moist suqar.

Ink stains can be removed by wetting the head of a sulfur tipped match and rubbing it on the spots. Rinse well. Rub warm milk into the hands each night, without rinsing, to get rid of any redness from these strong cleansers.

Brown Spots on the Hands

Called variously liver spots and old age spots, these round, splotchy brown marks so far have no medical explanation. And yet, they afflict and disturb most women and men anywhere in age from 30 or 40 and beyond. It has been suggested that this unattractive spotting of the skin indicates a toxic liver, laden with poisons. Linda Clark, in her book *Secrets of Natural Beauty* (Devin Adair), suggests a program of detoxification to get rid of brown spots.

This calls for drinking twice daily three tablespoons of liquid acidophilus plus one tablespoon of lactose or whey, mixed into eight ounces of water. To accompany this she suggests one tablespoon of desiccated liver daily or fresh liver served once a week.

Some creams purporting to remove brown spots from the skin have been found to contain ammoniated mercury. Because of the skin's ability to absorb good *and* bad topical applications, use of such a cream could cause mercury poisoning.

Warts

Warts are a common and very persistent affliction. Many times they are removed only to return again and again. Considered a viral infection, warts are also contagious, traveling as they do from one part of the body to another, and sometimes from one family member to another. A dermatologist can remove the warts and medicate the area. Other than that, Adelle Davis reports that an improved diet acids in wart disappearance, especially when vitamin A is emphasized.

Chapter 7

The Body Beautiful (Lower)

The feet, ankles, knees, legs, and thighs are usually sadly neglected when it comes to beauty care. And yet we are mighty dependent on these parts of our body for comfort in addition to attractiveness that can enhance our overall appearance.

How do you keep your feet and legs well and happy? You wiggle them around to get the fat off and keep them strong. Many a woman has taken ballet lessons not with an aim of artistic achievement, but to slim thick legs and trim her thighs. And who really cares that she was ungainly in her *pas de deux*? After a couple dozen lessons she will be superb in her bikini!

The Thighs

The thighs may be large and fatty even when the rest of the body is trim. There are many ways to reduce this area, but I find the practice of yoga the most beneficial because it exerts a toning action on the entire body. While the problem may appear to be localized in the upper thighs, if you are exercising sufficiently every day, and your diet is well planned, perhaps yoga is needed to help normalize glandular functions, which in turn could stabilize weight and prevent disproportionate gains. Yoga will stimulate the entire body and put it in better working condition.

While certain forms of exercise will aid particular areas of the body, the disciplined movements of Hatha yoga aid the body as a whole and increase its overall performance, even as they help to eliminate specific trouble areas. The following exercise should be beneficial in reducing thigh size. But a complete yoga plan would be of even greater advantage.

Seated on the floor, extend your legs in a straight line before you. Hold the knees straight and stretch your legs in a fan shape as far apart to either side as you can. Very slowly reach for your right foot with your right hand and your left foot with your left hand. You may not reach your feet on the first attempts, so do not force the movement. Slowly return to your original position. Repeat three or four times, or as long as it is comfortable.

Practiced over a period of time, this leg stretch should work at the rippled, fleshy thigh area and return better muscle tone to it.

Regular exercise is the most reliable way to tone and trim the thighs. Walking is excellent for both the upper and lower legs. Bicycling will also firm slack leg flesh. And if you're housebound, practice bicycling by lying on the floor, legs in the air, pedaling an imaginary bicycle.

In addition, try kneeling on the floor with your legs separated a bit. Very slowly ease the derrière down between your legs as they extend behind you, without using your hands for support. Repeat several times for effective thigh toning.

There are many women whose legs, especially the thighs, become laced over with tiny, thread-like veins. The condition is so unattractive that one hesitates to wear a bathing suit or shorts. A thick coverup base helps to conceal the spidery red veins, but this type of treatment is only temporary and cannot begin to solve the problem.

The eruption of tiny capillaries just under the skin is described by Dr. Thomas H. Sternberg, M.D., in his book *More Than Skin Deep* (Curtis Books, New York) as Cayenne Pepper Points, and is known among doctors as progressive pigmentary dermatosis. He says these pinpoint ruptures of the capillaries into the skin probably stem from a toxic effect on the capillaries, but the mechanism of origin is unknown. According to this doctor, some people with this ailment benefit from large doses of vitamin C and rutin.

Varicose Veins

Varicose veins are a major problem. They are uncomfortable, unsightly, and most unwelcome. You can have surgery to remove these veins, but after a period of relief, in some cases, they do reappear.

The circulatory problem that creates painful blockage of leg veins is medically treated by surgery and injection. Nutritionally, vitamins B, C and E are recommended for preventing and dissolving blood clots. According to Adelle Davis in *Let's Get Well*, some investigators believe faulty elimination to be a major cause of varicose veins, in that an overburdened bowel presses against the veins in the lower abdomen. This, in turn, is believed to break down the valves within the veins and allow a reverse blood flow.

Miss Davis suggests another cause of varicose veins to be a damaged liver, which would slow down the return of blood to the heart. This would be alleviated, she says, by a correct diet of wholegrain breads and cereals, fresh fruits, vegetables, meats, eggs, cheese, sour milk and nuts. In short, the exclusive consumption of unrefined foods, and the elimination of all processed foods from your diet.

Flaky Legs

Patches of dry, flaky skin afflict the legs of many women each winter. Commercial lotions and creams may not give enough aid, no matter how often they are applied. Stronger measures are needed to combat these stubborn patches of dry skin.

As you sit on the side of the bathtub, run warm water over your legs. Shake off the excess water and apply a good coating of blackstrap molasses or honey to the legs. This requires sitting for at least 30 minutes. You might choose to sit on a bath mat, or folded towel, and be armed with a book. After 30 minutes, rinse off the molasses and pat your legs dry. This application should be repeated daily until the condition clears up completely. If one time is effective, you might like to repeat the application either weekly or monthly to prevent its return.

A homemade lanolin cream can reinforce this treatment.

Melt together over hot water two tablespoons each of lanolin and olive oil. Mix thoroughly and massage into the dry leg areas. Only a very thin film is required, but this must be used each day until the situation clears up.

Alligator Knees

Rough knees are both uncomfortable and unattractive. If not given the proper attention, the knees can become so criss-crossed with lines as to resemble an alligator's back at times.

To work on those problem knees, start with almond meal.

Each day, wet your knees and scour them firmly with a hand-ful of meal (it's best to do this standing in the bathtub). Rinse them off, and while they are still moist, rub in a salad oil mixed with a few drops of apple cider vinegar. Blot dry and repeat.

Don't miss a day with this practice, and in a week or two your knees should be quite presentable.

Lanolin cream can be a help here, also, and since the area to be covered is so small, you can rub in the same cream you use for your flaky legs, blot off the excess, pull on your panty hose, and have the cream working for you all day.

Lumpy Knees

Unsightly lumps of flesh along the inner sides of the knees may defy all attempts to exercise them away. You may be in good physical condition and still have trouble reducing these unattractive bulges. If you are well exercised and know that the bulges are not excess poundage, the following exercise, recommended by an orthopedic physician for creating stronger knee muscles, might help tone those lumps of flesh.

Sitting comfortably in a chair, stretch one leg straight before you. Now curl the toes of the foot downward toward the sole of the foot, very slowly. Release the toes and relax the leg before repeating. Practice this movement several times, very slowly. Repeat the exercise with the other foot.

You can feel the slack muscles become taut if you place your fingers on the inner side of the knees. The exercise should become a daily practice, and be continued even after you notice improvement.

The squatting position in yoga is another beneficial exercise for toning the knees.

In a standing position, take a deep breath and go up on your toes. Exhale as you bend the knees and lower your body as far as possible, to try to sit on your heels. Inhale slowly and come up. In taking this position, you might find it necessary to hold onto a chair or table, or other support in order to maintain balance. Repeat as often as it is comfortable.

Thick Ankles

If your ankles are thick and seem to be too large in proportion to your legs, try this ankle exercise. If there is excess fat in this area, these invigorating and simple foot movements will help get rid of it.

Sit comfortably erect on a chair and hold your feet before you. Describe ten circles with each foot, going from right to left. Then reverse direction and roll your feet in the opposite direction.

Don't Ignore Your Feet

Fatigued and aching feet are often the price of a day's work. Even though you may not be overweight, your feet may become so tired that it is difficult to get through the evening.

Assuming you wear sensibly-heeled shoes, neither too high nor too flat, of a non-confining style, there are various exercises that can help strengthen the muscles of the foot and bring comfort. These exercises, though beneficial when practiced daily, are without value if you return to ill-fitting shoes for the major portion of your day. You can understand how a few minutes of care a day cannot possibly offset the long hours of poor posture and constricted foot movement brought about by the wrong size or shape of a shoe.

Did you know that you can use a rolling pin to exercise and relax your feet?

While seated in a chair, let your feet roll the pin back and forth from the toes to the heel, bearing down with a comfortable weight until you feel the increased stimulation in all parts of the foot.

Another foot-easer calls for you to lie flat on the floor with the soles of your feet propped against a wall. "Walk" the feet slowly up and down the wall, grasping at the wall with wide-spread toes. This open-toed movement brings cramped foot muscles into play and activates the blood circulation.

The Rocking Foot Balance is considered helpful in preventing flat feet, if used in conjunction with other good preventive practices.

For this exercise, sit in a squatting position with your weight on your toes. Slowly rock backward and come to rest flat on the feet. Slowly roll forward again, resting on the toes, and repeat these movements several times. If support is required, hold onto some stable object, the end of a bed perhaps, or a heavy chair.

Calluses

In our fashion conscious age, shoes are designed with style, not comfort, in mind. And every season, most of us run out to buy the latest in shoes to keep our wardrobes up to date. Although our shoes may reveal an eye for the newest styles, they can also cause us hours of discomfort. Most people suffer aggravating foot problems at least occasionally. Perhaps the most widespread complaint is calluses, those tough, hardened patches that can't usually be softened no matter how much cream we rub into them.

A visit to the podiatrist is probably the best thing you can do for calluses. Check your shoes to be sure they are well fitted. Squeezing feet into too-small shoes is one of the most impractical and painful habits one can develop. There is little pleasure to be had when the feet burn and ache from calluses.

A good foot bath of hot water and baking soda will sometimes help these hardened areas. After a good soaking, rub at the callused area with rough toweling and then apply a mixture of oil and vinegar; a teaspoon of vinegar to one-eight cup of oil. Rub in well and blot the excess. You can also use a pumice stone on the callused areas every day following your bath. Then rub in a nourishing cream or oil.

An unusual and quite pleasant way to treat callused feet is to keep a container of sand in your bathroom. After you've had your bath, put the container of sand in the bathtub and walk in place in it, up and down for about five minutes. This daily friction will aid a great deal with a callused foot problem. Rinse and dry the feet, and rub in a cream or oil before blotting.

Chapter 8

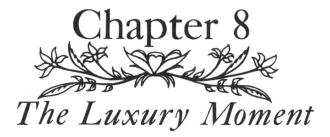

The Luxury Moment

Beauty baths have been part of daily life since long before Cleopatra took her famous milk dips. Perhaps the pinnacle of luxurious bathing was reached in Rome. Certainly the Romans showed every evidence of appreciating the benefits of a long, leisurely bath.

One Roman establishment, nearly 2,000 years ago, offered a choice of over 20 different types of baths. There were warm, hot, cold, fruit, vegetable, milk and honey baths—every type of exotic bathing experience imaginable.

I've seen the ruins of once magnificent bathing houses in Pompeii. Hot and cold ducts channeled the desired temperature of water to spacious marble pools. Huge urns contained a wide variety of sweet-smelling oils, pomades, lotions and herbal unguents which were rubbed into the bather's body before he took to the water, and again when he emerged.

The baths in Pompeii were near the marketplace and halls of business. Shopkeepers, craftsmen and politicians alike could saunter to the baths for a respite from their day's labors, or even for a bit of wheeling and dealing in business much as is done today in various clubs.

According to biographers of French courtesan Ninon

de L'Enclos, the fountain of youth did indeed lie in water. Ninon, who remained youthful and enticing well into her seventies revelled in a bath of herbs that kept her vigorous and attractive long after her contemporaries had turned in their paint boxes and false curls.

So we can see that bathing is all it's been held to be during centuries past; a relaxing, invigorating and pleasant way to restore energy to a fatigued body, soothe jangled nerves, and bring clear thought to a frantic mind.

I once knew a woman who said when all else failed her, when she could not reason with an annoyed husband, her children became impossible, her checking account was overdrawn, or she found the world unbearable, she took a bath. A long, leisurely bath, that unwound her coiled emotions and held her in its warm embrace.

She would lock the bathroom door and become an alchemist over the tub as she prepared the brew that would restore her peace of mind. When she emerged from her bath she found she could cope with her problems to a surprisingly effective degree.

There is no great secret here, for balneology, the science of using water for its curative powers, has been a part of the medical world for a long time. And even if the ailment is no more than a tense, tired body, a penetrating bath can restore serenity. This, too, is a form of healing.

European belief in the efficacy of bathing for health far exceeds our own. I have visited water spas around the world, and have never been disappointed in the multitude of different baths they offer.

Here in America we do have some institutions promoting the benefits of bathing in hot spring waters and sulfur waters, or offering baths of another nature. But some of these places promote their golf courses as much as their baths, and it seems to me they should be able to attract people by virtue of the calming, restorative values of their waters alone, instead of having to compete with places of amusement.

The worth of mineral baths appears to lie in the fact that the body is encouraged to heal itself by absorbing helpful minerals from the water. That belief is certainly not far-fetched, for correction of any body ailment takes place when the body rallies and overcomes its own disturbance. Even medical people would not say that medicine heals, but rather, that it permits the ailing body to cure itself.

The bath should be a deliberate undertaking, whether you are using it to calm and restore yourself or merely to cleanse your body. A quick dousing and drying can in no way be equated with a bath of longer length and more attentive preparation, for the results are entirely different.

When you concoct your very own beauty baths, let your imagination run wild. Use the abundance of materials growing in your garden, waiting on the grocer's shelves, or available from a botanical supply house. Anything you toss into the tub that has nutritional, stimulating, cleansing or relaxing qualities will reward both your body and spirits.

Preparing Your Bath

In preparing for a bath, it is good to remember that the need to bathe is greater today than ever before. When Cleopatra lolled in her swan-shaped tub, and Marie Antoinette enjoyed her gilded bath, pollution of the air was practically unknown. These beautiful women bathed for freshness and luxury.

Nowadays, with the air heavily laden with particles of dirt and soot, radioactive fallout, and poisonous sprays, bathing is a vital necessity. It is the only way we can remove the external collection of toxins that gather on our sensitive skins.

Never rush your bath. Set aside a time for complete peace and relaxation during the bath. In fact, rest and bathing can be successfully combined to produce excellent results you could not get from rest alone.

The time of bathing depends upon the individual, and should be chosen for convenience. Once begun, the bath should be approached and anticipated as a daily pleasure, rather than a chore.

One woman I know takes her long, deep bath at midnight, after her family responsibilities are completed.

"At that hour," she says, "I'm free. I look forward to my bath as others might look forward to a dinner out, or the theatre or a movie."

Another friend prefers an early morning bath. She works outside her home, so she arises an hour earlier than she would ordinarily and luxuriates in her tub of scented water, readying herself for a serene approach to a busy day in the business world.

"Nighttimes," she says, "I take a shower, not too stimulating, but refreshing. But I much prefer to start the day in beauty and serenity than to lose the glory of such a bath by going to bed, and to sleep."

Those are their methods. You will find the time most suitable for you, but the long, soothing bath is a joy, and once enjoyed, easily becomes a habit.

Bath water should never be too cold or too hot. Yoga teaches that the body should never be shocked. Sudden plunges into a "brisk" shower or "hot tub" are a brutal jolt to the body. A shower that starts out hot and then changes quickly to cold is also damaging. The resultant violent reactions of the nervous system can never be beneficial.

Water should be comfortably warm. Showers should have the same temperature from start to finish. Having chosen your convenient time, when there will be no interruptions to your relaxing beauty bath, fill the tub, having everything at hand that you will need. Experiment, vary your bath, and discover a new experience.

What's Wrong with Soap?

Most of us were reared with the echo of "Cleanliness is next to Godliness," so that daily use of soap on our bodies is second nature. But it is known, even if not spoken of too often, that the mania among many Americans for antiseptic body cleanliness has probably done more harm than good when the daily bathing ritual includes a bar of alkaline soap. And this happens to be especially true if that soap is one of the highly publicized germ-killing deodorant soaps.

Soap making is believed to have been a by-product of early Roman sacrifices, when animals put to the blaze left ashes and a bit of fat. Rain mixing with these sacrificial remains caused suds to form. The Bible, too, speaks of using soap, so it is a long established practice, and one not easy to forego. Yet excessive use of an alkaline soap will often cause irritated skin and eczema resulting from the skin's acid mantle being too often disturbed and not permitted to replace itself.

Today's soap is essentially the metallic salt of a fatty acid coming from animal or vegetable fats, and is produced by the action of caustic alkali on these same fats. Added to the resultant product may be coloring agents, antioxidants, perfume, and in the case of medicated or deodorant soaps, antimicrobials. Five germ killers were recently listed by the Food and Drug Administration as "not generally regarded as safe for incorporation into toilet bars for personal hygienic use."

Unless you are involved in heavy industrial work, or an occupation in which the skin comes in contact with sooty and oily substances, there are skin cleansers which will work far more effectively than the usual bar of soap. At the same time, the substitutes will not produce the drying, roughening effects of soap.

If you feel you are not really clean unless you wash with a bar of soap, don't despair. A few manufacturers apparently feel the same way, and have placed their non-alkaline soap on the market. One brand I know of contains oatmeal and bran, and tests out with a pH compatible to the skin. Another well-known brand combines protein with its cleansing qualities, and also has a pH comparable to skin. So be willing to scout around for your soap rather than toss a few bars into your basket at the supermarket. The little bit of extra effort certainly pays off.

Scented Soaps

There is a multitude of new soaps on the market, scented in fresh fruit fragrances, and colored to match. But beware: the synthetic scents and dyes that lace the current crop of soaps haven't been any closer to an orchard than the laboratory where they were formulated. And the chemical additives used to "flavor" this mockery of a natural product will create problems for many people sensitive to the laboratory-created fruit soaps.

High Class Cleansers

You can add a touch of luxury to your bath when you combine one-fourth cup of cornmeal and the same amount of powdered orris root. Drop the mixture into a cotton bag or square, secure the ends, and scrub away.

Cornmeal as a bath additive offers cleansing, friction-producing action to slough off dead skin cells. And the sweet smelling orris root will remind you of spring violets.

For another elegant bath, use a mixture of almond meal, powdered elderflower blossoms and cornmeal. Tie up the ingredients in a cotton bag or square, and use it as a wash-cloth. Your skin will be left soft, scented, and beautifully clean, with a slight residue of nutrients to give you a head start in skin care.

Cleansers from Nature

Then, of course, for those who want to pursue nature in her own ways, search out supplies of the soapwort, or Bouncing Bet as we know it in America, soapbark and soapberry plants, or the flowering heads of the sweet pepper bush. These plants all produce a substance known as saponin, which lathers in water. All were used by American Indians and early pioneers as acceptable and harmless cleansers. Botanical supply houses carry some of these items, but it might be wise to test your skin's reaction to the plants before having an overall ablution.

In those remote areas of Colombia where yucca grows profusely, I saw village women produce a cleansing agent from the versatile yucca plant, which also provided food for their families, and fibers for string, rope, paper, woven baskets, and even clothing. To create an acceptable cleanser, yucca roots are chopped and macerated in water.

Types of Baths

Bathing practices differ around the world, and take on a variety of different forms. Japan has her communal or family pools. The Scandinavians relish a steaming sauna followed by a plunge into a cold lake, or pool. Once, on a visit to Stockholm in late November, I decided to experience for myself the sensation of full sauna bathing. But I stopped short of the plunge down the hill from the warm sauna house when I saw the frozen lake.

There are many famous baths in Germany that have been frequented for a couple of centuries. Baden-Baden offers a memorable mud bath, the benefits of which I suspect stem from the minerals in the flowing black soil with which I found myself plastered during my visit there.

Gathering information on spas around the world proved to be one of the most enjoyable assignments I've ever had. However, it almost proved my undoing in the charming, old-world village of Bad Neuenahr, in the German Rhineland. Bad Neuenahr is famous for its natural mineral water and mud baths, and in the evenings the band performs in the beautiful concert hall. You can promenade through sculptured gardens, down white gravel walks, and stop at each fountain to sip the naturally carbonated water splashing down over lava rocks from the nearby mountains.

Arrangements for my bath were made in a mixture of French and English, for my German is limited to a couple of words. And the same applied to the director's French and English. Nevertheless, I entered a sumptuous room with an attendant who wheeled in a steaming bucket of mud. Hildegaard was generous with the applications and shortly, I was rolled up into a rubberized blanket, imprisoned and helpless. I found this was not the time to change my mind about a mud bath, for not only could I not communicate verbally, I couldn't even get my hands free.

Mud baths are a great leveler. After time was allowed

for my skin to absorb the minerals from the thick, dark mud I was wearing, Hildegaard unwrapped me and motioned me into a sunken tub, and turned a hose on me. A great deal of dignity goes down the drain along with the mud.

Next I was led to a thermal pool, which contained an assortment of men and women cavorting around. In I plunged, expecting to swim, but this turned out to be an exercising group, and eager bathers tried to explain in sign language that I was to follow their lead and perform on the various bars and loops within the pool as the director called out instructions. In German, of course.

Thirty minutes of this and I was exhausted, though these regular bathers were lustily executing turns and rolls in the water. Each time I tried to leave, the bathers seemed under the impression I didn't understand, and hauled me back for more. I think I might have drowned from exhaustion if I hadn't finally broken away and escaped by swimming underwater to the pool's edge. I don't think I stopped running until I reached the dressing room. I am still impressed by the fact that the men and women in that pool were in their sixties, seventies and eighties. I didn't know whether to attribute the feeling of elation that remained with me for several days to the rich minerals in both mud and water, or to my narrow escape.

Another city that drew me to its baths was Budapest. There, on a hillside in the historic city of Buda that is separated from its sister city of Pest by the Danube, one can lounge in sequestered splendor in mineral waters favored by the long ago Queen of Hungary.

However, as exotic as these mineral baths may be, you can have a luxury bath in your own bathroom.

Mineral Bath

Dissolve a pound of epsom salts in a tub of warm water. For the next 15 to 20 minutes, alternately massage your body and relax. Towel yourself dry energetically to produce a fair amount of friction. This type of bath leaves you with a sense of well-being, and also has a beneficial effect on sore muscles or any stiffness of the body.

One nutritionist I know recommends the epsom salts bath as a means of aiding the body in the removal of toxins through the skin. The epsom salts bath shouldn't be taken too frequently; it is more in the nature of a restorative for overworked muscles and ligaments.

Salt Bath

A similar bath can be prepared using a salt water solution. Remember the invigorating feeling after a swim in the ocean? It's not just all that fresh air; it has to come also from the minerals in the water. Try it at home. Use up to one pound of salt in the tub, according to how much surf you want. For the best results, use sea salt rather than regular table salt.

Nourishing Baths

We are all aware that nourishing masks are great for the face, but we mustn't forget that the rest of the body needs nourishment, too. A bath is one of the nicest ways to do this.

Milk Bath

A milk bath is a great treat for your body. Thirsty pores will be saturated with this calcium covering and the results will be a firmer but beautifully soft skin.

There has been revived interest in milk bathing recently.

So much so that many cosmetic companies have included lovely packets of sweetly scented "milk" powders in their lines. However, the preservatives and other chemicals added to what might once have been milk makes a bath in this type of solution of questionable value. These cosmetic milk baths can cost as much as four dollars for six ounces, but the woman who wants to bathe in milk can buy it for far less in the supermarket—about 31 cents for the same amount.

Oil Rub

Another delightful body treatment is a vigorous oil rub with a nourishing salad oil. Just before taking your bath, spread a towel on the floor to stand on. Massage in generous quantities of oil all over. Sit down and read for 15 minutes. Start running your bath and take the back of a butter knife (do not use a sharp bladed knife) to remove the excess oil. Even a spoon handle will do. Run this over your body, starting with your legs, and work all the way upward. Remove the excess oil from the spoon with paper toweling. Then step into the tub of hot water and proceed with your regular bath. Rub vigorously with a towel to remove any last vestiges of excess oil. And do be careful while in the tub, for this is a luxurious but slippery bath. Your skin, afterwards, will be as soft and luscious as a baby's.

Vinegar Bath

Although it's not glamorous, the down-to-earth vinegar bath can be very helpful in relieving aching muscles or itching skin, when the itching is due to a lack of acid on the body. Pour one cup of apple cider vinegar into your tub of warm water. Soak for 15 or 20 minutes and allow the vinegar and water to soothe both skin and body.

Oil Baths

The oil bath answers many needs. First of all, we abuse our skins by subjecting them to the assaults of detergents, chemicals, dyes from clothing, and similar harsh substances. In addition, heavy doses of sunshine, harsh winds and cold air do their damage. Bathing in an emulsion of oil and water helps to restore some of the moisture we tend to lose, especially as we grow older.

There is little to compare with the comfort on a winter's day of sinking back into a brimming tub laced with sweetly scented oil. Our dry bodies seem to open their pores in response to this soothing treatment. The soft film of oil on the water clings to the skin, and even after a brisk toweling, enough oil remains to make one feel more lithe and supple, because the dryness of the outer layer of skin has been lessened.

The day after such a bath, the benefits are still with us. Our feet feel smooth within our shoes, and we seem to glide as we walk.

Although there are preparations on the market for an infinite variety of oil baths, from perfumed liquids to marble-like pellets that dissolve in the water, we can also make our own, to be sure that we are getting no undesirable mineral oil in our baths. This by-product of crude oil does not soothe the skin; on the contrary, it leaves deposits in the opened pores which can cause irritation. It is always far better to use organic matter for, in, and on the body, in preference to any chemical.

Herbal Bath Oil

For those who like a smooth, silky feeling, and who want to experiment with homemade oils, try mixing one cup of any vegetable or nut oil, with one tablespoon of herbal or castile shampoo. Add several drops of rose oil for a pleasantly scented mixture.

If you have a blender, set it at the highest speed, then whip the mixture to a froth to emulsify the solution. Or, beat with an egg beater until well blended. Bottle the oil, and use four tablespoons to a tub of water. Pour it into the warm water and swish it about before stepping in and luxuriating. Massage your body under water to derive the fullest benefits from this delightful coating.

Herbal Baths

In treating yourself to herbal baths, remember that while an occasional addition to your tub may be very pleasant, for lasting results such baths should be taken weekly over a period of about two months. Then, according to your needs or whims, you can switch to another type of bath.

From the Kitchen

For a soothing bath add rosemary, sage, or any herb of the mint family to the water. Prepare the herbs in a dish of hot water before straining into the bath. You might also wish to make small gauze bags to hang over the tub faucet, in order to have sweet scents available without the regular brewing.

For these small bags, simply sew a square large enough to hold a handful of any crushed mixture you choose of dried flowers, or herbs and pungent grasses. Lace a drawstring into the top of the bag, pull the top together and tie. As the water from the faucet pours down, it will carry the fragrance of the bath bag into your tub.

From the Garden

There are many, many refreshing herbal and floral baths. The variety is as large as your garden and your imagination.

Gather a quantity of leaves, petals, herbs and roots to have on hand, and use them either separately or combined. You might like to grow some of these items, or order them from an herbalist.

I've a friend who arranged an incredibly beautiful area of bath herbs and flowers around her small terrace. Visitors are always enchanted with an invitation to lunch, or to have a casual visit, when they are seated on the terrace and can inhale the mingled aromas of resinous, sweet and pungent plants. Though Ann also uses some of her plants for cooking and scenting, I remember best the fragrant balm, the rose geranium, and the nostalgic lightness of lavender, all put to good use in the bath.

When you are ready for a fragrant bath, steep a cupful of the mixed petals and leaves in a pint of boiling water for about 15 minutes. Strain the liquid and pour into your tub.

From Wild Plants

Or you might try the wild herbs that are so plentiful and easy to come by. Plantain leaves, when thoroughly dried and crumbled into a large bowl with scalding water poured over them, make an excellent addition to a bath. Steep the brew for 20 minutes or so, then strain into your tub of warm water. For the best results, it is suggested that you bathe in this solution several times a week. Use a fresh solution each time, of course. That requires a lot of plantain picking, but it's well worth the effort. Juliette de Bairacli Levy, the renowned herbalist, suggests bathing with plantain for skin ailments, too.

Blackberry leaves, dried and crumbled in the manner described above, then steeped and strained into the tub make another old herbal bath that is supposed to invigorate the body.

Anyone who is fortunate enough to have her own raspberry patch knows the great value of this remarkable plant. These berries are fast disappearing from the commercial market because of the labor involved in picking them, and the perishable nature of the fruit. A wise gardener would add a couple of bushes to her plot to avail herself of both fruit and leaves. As a fruit, the raspberry is considered a nervine and general tonic, and the excellent astringent qualities of the dried leaves make them a cleansing and refreshing addition to the bath.

Dry Baths

I learned of the *gant de massage,* or massage glove, in Paris. The proprietor of a small shop became quite excited reciting the marvelous benefits of brushing away at the body without benefit of water. He said one could have a body as polished as the finest marble, though with a great deal more life, if the friction glove was used frequently.

And as for suffering from insomnia, ah, madame! Those days will be over for the insomniac who arises during a sleepless night, removes his clothing and proceeds to apply the glove in even strokes from the bottoms of his feet to his head.

And it really works! All those Frenchmen (and Frenchwomen) can't be wrong, for from the amount of friction gloves sold in Paris alone (they're sold all over town), I'd say there was a lot of dry bathing going on.

I use the friction glove in place of a washcloth daily, on all parts of the body below the neck, in my bath. I have, on a sleepless night or two, applied to my body the long, slow strokes of the rough-textured aloe-brush I keep especially for this purpose. And I've fallen asleep shortly afterward.

Don't exert pressure when you use the friction glove. Light strokes will do it.

Internal Bathing

Another area of bathing that is of special concern to women is internal hygiene. Chemical douches are undesirable and not very helpful. Toni Stabile, in her well documented book, *Cosmetics, The Great American Skin Game,* reports that American women were expected to spend $35 to $45 million in one year for feminine hygiene sprays, and quoted Dr. Alan F. Guttmacher as saying he saw no need for these sprays.

Yet all of us like to feel fresh, and it is not easy to resist the hard-sell commercials that show daisies and roses sifting down upon the woman who has a container of the touted spray in her hand. But from the point of view of effectiveness and safety, you would be far better advised to prepare your own solution.

A mild infusion of rosemary, carefully strained, can be used for its clean, aromatic scent. Other herbs also serve nicely in douches that are cleansing and refreshing at the same time. Mint water can be used alone or combined with other herbs. Rose geranium leaves steeped in water and added to the douche water can prove far more pleasant than artificially scented commercial preparations. You can also use apple cider vinegar for another refreshing solution.

Deodorants

Many of us find that aluminum-based deodorants irritate the sensitive underarm area. Anyone with this problem should switch to a non-chemical deodorant which will not stop the normal discharge of perspiration, but will eliminate the developing odor, and which will be more acceptable to your skin.

To make your own deodorant, use a lettuce leaf extract produced by bruising the leaf and squeezing a drop of chlorophyll from the mangled leaf. The heavier the type of lettuce, the more successful this will be. Try for a sturdy romaine; avoid iceberg lettuce—it will not work at all.

Mash and bruise the dark green part of the leaf and allow a drop of chlorophyll to fall into your palm. Spread the liquid on the underarm area and let it dry.

You'll find this a wonderful deodorant as the chlorophyll in the leaf destroys the bacteria which cause perspiration odor. In the summertime and fall, the chrysanthemum leaf is even superior to the lettuce leaf for preventing odor.

You might also like to try just a drop of lavender oil in the underarm area. It is quite helpful in eliminating odor.

Talcum Powders

Some dusting powders and talcums contain boric acid which, when taken into the body (as it can be through chafed skin) is capable of causing internal damage. According to Charles Perry, the English nutritionist and beautician, boric acid should be avoided in any form. This may be difficult, because it is sometimes used as an emulsifier in vanishing and cold creams.

However, you might try ordering pure talcum from your pharmacist. It is scentless, but without harmful ingredients. Be sure to specify *pure*. Fuller's Earth, though not the appealing white of dusting powder, is another harmless covering. Or try rice powder, sifted until it is fluffy and free of any sediment. This was a popular face powder until the turn of the century.

Chapter 9

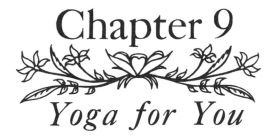

Yoga for You

A Western version of this Eastern system of mental and physical exercise grows more and more popular with Americans because of its ease of performance and moderate pace. I have seen older men and women regain better usage of their bodies after faithfully practicing yoga movements daily. And young people who have slipped into a sedentary life style before turning to yoga exercises actually blossom when they practice these sensible body movements.

One of the most exciting and rewarding things ever to happen to me was my introduction to yoga. This discipline, adapted to the Western world, has sustained my interest like none of the other forms of exercise I have tried from time to time. Did it change my life? Indeed it did. Both physically and mentally, daily performance of these simple body movements has increased my health, vigor, and mental outlook. If that sounds like a testimonial, it is a testimonial based on fact.

I first learned of yoga while living in France. A group of employees at the American Embassy in Paris decided to fight the effects of their well-provisioned cafeteria and sedentary office positions (which might have made them privy to interesting events in a fascinating city, but didn't do a thing for their pulpy figures). They engaged an Indian instructor and formed a yoga class. I was not impressed until two friends in the group began to display figures I never imagined them capable of.

I observed that not only did yoga work wonders on the figure, but just as important, it seemed to sweep away mental cobwebs and invest its proponents with a keen zest for living.

Upon returning to the States to live, I sought out a yoga class and was fortunate enough to find myself under the tutelage of Joy Gorin. Ms. Gorin teaches in an unhurried manner, and has introduced thousands of students to a new and quite wonderful way of life.

Practicing yoga daily, old irritations slipped away, compassionate thinking took hold, and a vast reserve of energy enabled me to work long, rewarding hours without tiring. The freedom and serenity generated by a well exercised body are almost indescribable. One learns to cope effectively with seemingly impossible situations.

Things that would once have sent me into a tailspin are now bearable, and usually can be solved. This kind of capability is accomplished by putting one's own feelings beyond the reach of petty irritants.

One yoga student advised me to learn to remain calm in the face of small disasters and to save my panic for larger ones. The clever logic behind this philosophy is that the discipline that comes from remaining calm during minor crises gradually increases our confidence and diminishes the impact of each annoying or disconcerting event. And the healthy, well adjusted mind deeply influences the body.

One of the great values of practicing yoga comes from the controlled slowness with which one learns to move his body in this discipline. This controlled approach develops agility and a litheness of movement. There should never be pressure to learn a certain position or exercise, but instead, a dedication and determination to be in command of the body eventually, without resorting to force. This will restore grace and incredible fitness to all who persevere, and who do not rush. For yoga is not as beneficial if the postures are attained too quickly.

There are several facets of yoga which fall into two basic approaches—mental and physical. The mental disciplines are concerned with study, knowledge, devotion and meditation. We are primarily concerned here with physical, or Hatha, yoga, which involves regulated body movements leading to the attainment of various postures, or *asanas*.

Why Is Yoga Better?

Though most body movements that keep the body supple and youthful are desirable, it is my feeling that many calisthenic type exercises are too demanding. Very few people have a daily exercise plan; most are starters and stoppers. And when your body is not in top shape and you begin exerting it with demanding movements, there is a possibility of damage, from strained muscles or dislocation.

Unlike calisthenic types of exercise, yoga offers gentle, easy body movements that can be performed at almost any age. Everyone can benefit from some yoga exercise.

This is not to say that yoga is the only kind of exercise I advocate. There are many other excellent activities, like swimming and walking. I simply feel that anything that exhausts or puts undue strain on the body is not advisable, especially after the age of 30.

Yoga Teachers

One of the unfortunate aspects of yoga classes is that some teachers may attempt to push beginners into advanced postures too quickly, causing strain and injury to unexercised muscles. There are no rules or regulations governing yoga teachers in most areas. Many former students will complete a ten week course and announce they are forming their own class, when a much longer involvement of study and practice is required. A sincere and dedicated teacher realizes the importance of a thorough knowledge of the body and its limitations, the need to approach body movements with caution and the workings of the body as related to physical exercise.

It is vital to work only with a qualified instructor, and this will require checking around, also inquiring about the teacher's involvement in yoga. And it would be helpful to interview some of the teacher's former students.

My own instructor, some years ago, taught me the great value of an unhurried approach to yoga exercising. Joy Gorin has instilled in all her students the need to move the body slowly and gently toward its idealization. So I shared her teachings in my own book on yoga, *Look Younger, Look Prettier* (Rodale, 1972), instructing readers that greater benefits come from slow and steady practice rather than a rush to perfect a movement.

Yoga Brings Peace and Beauty

Yogic principles in themselves are beautiful, just to hear. Peace within oneself, no harsh self-condemnation, but a sincere attempt to correct any faults and to know the truth about oneself, and a desire to develop greater serenity are just some of the aims. A positive approach to and belief in life is another attitude to be developed.

As for bringing peace and beauty to someone who takes to heart its precepts, it is all quite easy. It isn't so much what you add to your life as what you remove from it. Inner peace comes with the awareness that much of our day is devoted to struggle and acquisition, and the realization that our needs are much less than we think.

Beauty is inherent in everyone. Haste, impatience, tension and bitterness stamp themselves on their victims and remove this beauty. By practicing yoga, one breathes more deeply, thereby relaxing and growing more serene and attractive. And flexing the body in the various physical exercises helps it to function better and remain vigorously youthful.

Yoga and Diet

Total involvement in yoga is closely related to dietary habits. Yoga can help you only as far as you want to be helped. While it is good to perform health-giving physical movements that create an agile body, if you feed that body inferior foods at the same time, you are limiting the full benefits of yoga. The foods that Westerners practicing yoga are advised to consume are those that are wholesome, fresh and unprocessed.

You need not be a vegetarian to practice yoga. Yoga benefits can be enjoyed by meat eaters as well as vegetarians. Those striving for the highest yogic precepts may eventually turn toward vegetarianism, though.

Breathing Techniques

A great benefit of yoga is found in the special type of controlled deep breathing, called the Complete Breath, which accompanies the Hatha system of body movements.

Regular breathing, the way you and I inhale every day, is generally shallow, not fully expanding or completely removing waste from the lungs.

Complete breathing requires long, slow inspiration of oxygen, pushing the indrawn air into the furthermost reaches of the lungs by expanding the stomach area. The chest is not forced out, for this would limit the oxygen intake.

Yogic breathing should be practiced at specific times only, otherwise you will hyperventilate, or take in too much oxygen and experience a sensation of lightheaded giddiness. Yogic breathing should never completely replace regular breathing.

These deeply indrawn breaths come in handy early in the morning when they serve to get the circulation going. They are also beneficial when practicing yoga exercises, or other forms of exercise. They serve as a calming agent when you are frightened, unnerved, angry, or experiencing any extreme emotion which, generally, causes your breathing to become shallow and rapid. A few slow abdomen-deep breaths will flood fresh oxygen through your body and help to stabilize your emotions.

When you fill your lungs with fresh air, you cause your bloodstream to pump its cleansing action throughout your body. This in turn helps to clear out impurities and bring a renewed color to your skin. Deep breathing is also referred to as beauty breathing because of this action.

Alternate breathing is another valuable breathing technique. This is the process of breathing through one nostril at a time, or alternately between the two. It is used to compose the mind, to gain a more serene sense of self and, in addition, can help open stuffy or blocked nasal passages.

Most Hatha movements are practiced on the floor. So for alternate breathing, sit erect on the floor with your legs in a comfortable tailor fashion. Place the ends of your index and middle fingers just above your nose against your forehead. Rest your right thumb against the right nostril, without pressure. Your ring finger will rest lightly against the left nostril and the little finger against it.

Expel all the air from your lungs through both nostrils, then close the right nostril by pressing your right thumb against it. Breathe deeply through the left nostril to fill the lungs to a count of eight.

Close the left nostril by pressing the ring finger onto it. Hold your breath for a count of four, then open the right nostril by removing your thumb, and expel the air through the nostril to a count of eight.

Keep the left nostril closed. To a count of eight, deep breathe through the right nostril. Press both nostrils closed to the count of four before removing your ring finger from the left nostril and exhaling to a count of eight.

Do this only a few times each day.

Yoga and Insomnia

Insomniacs can find great relief in yoga. After years of taking barbiturates or sedatives to induce sleep, the insomniac becomes convinced that he needs pills to put him to sleep. If you are one of these, you *can* give them up. First you have to know why you aren't sleeping. Coffee or tea can keep you awake for hours. Or if you allow yourself to become tense, and you maintain that level of disturbance in the evening, chances are you will not be able to fall asleep with any ease.

This is knowing your problem. The second step is wanting to overcome it.

Yoga will help you transcend both problems. With your first lesson in yoga, usually instruction in a rolling movement of the body on the floor, you begin to relieve tensions. As you progress in these body movements you will learn stretching positions that bring total relaxation to uptight bodies, and which prepare you for restful sleep. A well-exercised body and a serene mind are the most potent tranquilizers.

One woman told me that when she cannot fall asleep, or awakens in the middle of the night, she gets out of bed and practices the basic rolling exercise, and can then fall asleep when she returns to bed.

This is a wonderfully relaxing exercise to perform anytime you are tense and nervous.

Sit on the floor in loose clothing—no belts or shoes. Gather your knees in your arms and tuck your head down toward the knees. Slowly roll forward, then backward until your back is on the floor, then forward again. Keep your body in motion for several rolls.

Yoga and Smoking

The discipline and self awareness that come with the practice of yoga can help you to alter undesirable habits, like smoking, you had not the willpower to change before. Deep breathing when you want a cigarette can substitute admirably for the deeply indrawn smoking action. In the beginning, deep breathing may only delay you from lighting a cigarette. But as you practice this cleansing, restorative breathing technique you should lose your desire for tobacco altogether. Coupled with the physical movements of yoga, deep breathing will also calm jangled nerves, which a cigarette cannot do safely.

Yoga During Pregnancy

There are many yoga exercises that can help prepare your body for an easier delivery. All exercises that stress flexing and limbering the muscles of the legs and pelvic area should be of great help to the expectant mother.

The squatting exercise will accustom the body to the eventual position of the actual birth process. And interestingly enough, obviously knowledgeable primitive women give birth in this manner, without benefit of a hospital bed.

To perform this exercise, stand upright and breathe deeply as you rise on your toes. Exhale as you come down, and continue to descend until you reach a seated position on your heels. Rest your hands lightly on your knees and remain in this position only a few moments in the beginning. Gradually increase the time to two or three minutes. Then return to an upright position by rising on your toes and dropping your heels to the floor.

Another effective exercise is to kneel on the floor with your knees apart. Grasp your heels behind you with your hands, and slowly lower your derrière to the space between your feet. If you don't reach the floor on your first attempt, slowly elevate the hips and then try again. This movement will develop flexibility in the pelvic area.

Exercising at the Office

Many people with interesting office jobs find that by mid-afternoon, after several hours of intense concentration, they are physically exhausted. Remember that your body can become tired from lack of exercise as well as from physical exertion.

Assuming your health is good and your daytime fatigue stems from a lack of planned movement (which you should *plan* to do at home), here are two yoga exercises that can be quite refreshing and invigorating to a body in need of a mid-day toning.

Take a deep breath that goes all the way to the abdomen, as you stand in an upright position. Lift the arms overhead and lightly clasp the hands together. Center the head within the almost straight arms. Very slowly, stretching the body from the waist upward, bend sideways to the right, keeping the head within the arms, and holding the arms as straight as possible.

Swing very slowly in this sideways movement on toward the feet, breathing in and out as you do so. Without pause, slowly swing on around to the left side of the body until you return to your starting position with the arms overhead. By now you have completed a full circle that has carried the body sideways, downward, sideways on the rise, and around to return to a tall position.

Now repeat this movement in the opposite direction, swinging slowly to the left, rotating to the right, then standing upright once again.

This movement calls on unused muscles and pulls them into invigorating play to really stimulate the chair-weary body. It can be practiced as many times a day as you choose, and is easy enough to perform beside your desk, or in the lounge.

Another good stretcher for the lower part of your body requires you to stand upright with your feet flat on the floor. Take a deep breath and slowly lift one knee toward your chest. Reach with both hands for the knee and slowly bring it up and inward to rest as close to the chest as possible. Deep breathe in and out. Release your hold on the knee and allow it to return to the floor.

Repeat this exercise with the other leg.

Practicing this one several times quickens circulation to give you a lift. But do not perform beyond a point of comfort, and do not force the knee toward the chest. Guide and support it as far as it will go without strain.

Toning the Face

Practicing toning exercises, especially for the face, requires the use of a cream to lubricate the skin. Stretching dry skin with facial grimaces only brings additional grief. Before starting your facial movements, carefully massage in with the fingertips a softening cream. This will prevent undue tightening of the skin and make it more pliable.

When you àre alone, try practicing The Lion for excellent facial stimulation. Muscles in both the face and throat receive a toning from the exaggerated expressions of this exercise.

Sit on your heels and place your hands on your knees. Breathe deeply and tense your back. Thrust your hands out before you and spread your fingers in a stiffened fan shape. Stick your tongue out and down as far as possible and force the eyes wide open and look upward. Hold your body in this stiff position for a few moments, then exhale and relax.

The Lotus Is Not for Beginners

Many people associate the practice of yoga with the lotus position, and when they find themselves unable to assume this difficult posture they decide that yoga is not for them. But inability to perform the lotus is no cause for despair.

You will be able to make your body more flexible by constant practice. Few people can gain these advanced positions right away. Do not use force or become impatient. Yoga teaches the value of avoiding haste. Work toward the ideal rather than forcing an unprepared body into difficult positions. The ideal here would be to limber your hip area. And try to remember that it probably took a long time for your body to become stiff and intractable; so you must allow a portion of that time to resurrect it.

To limber the hip area in order to gain the agility needed for the lotus position, sit on the floor and extend your left leg before you. Bend the knee of your right leg and place the right ankle on the left thigh. Very gently place your right hand on the right knee and start rocking it to the floor and back without stopping. Rhythmically push down as though bouncing a ball. Change legs after a while and repeat.

Persistence in this movement will also whittle down the hips.

Yoga Is for Everybody

Some of us who have led sedentary lives desire some form of exercise as we grow older, but fear putting undue strain on our hearts. Dr. Lawrence E. Lamb, consultant to the Director of Life Science for the National Aeronautics and Space Administration, has said that the cause of coronary artery disease in adults is traceable to underdeveloped hearts.

Exercise is one of the best ways to enlarge the heart, he advises. Physical conditioning is also helpful in reducing blood cholesterol levels. So for beauty and health, I would heartily endorse yoga as a moderate approach to a necessary daily activity.

Chapter 10

Pounds in Problem Places

Women who have successfully dieted off unwanted pounds experience a great sense of accomplishment. But disappointment follows quickly on the heels of elation if the skin does not regain its former elasticity and instead, hangs in folds after the fat is gone. Dieting and exercise must always be an inseparable duo if you want to be a sylph instead of a sack. Women all over the world write me of their dissatisfaction after a substantial weight loss, when they have not increased their physical activity to help tighten the skin while dieting.

In Sweden I have seen men and women exercising at off moments in the day. Waiting for a traffic light, running along the road between bus stops, and in the rest rooms of department stores. And their stunning figures! As the French say: *Regardez!*

I firmly believe we Americans are finally becoming aware of the dangers of obesity, the need to correct our excessive food consumption, and the attendant need to exercise. It is a hungry world we live in, and gluttony should no more have a place in it than violence or any other form of willful destruction. Combining moderation in food habits with daily exercise, our nation can become the country that minimizes illness and maximizes health.

Why Diet?

Perhaps looks aren't everything, but health is. The Metropolitan Life Insurance Company warns that for every inch your waist measurement exceeds your chest measurement, you can subtract two years from your life.

Since overweight is usually attributable to overeating you might like to follow the advice of Dr. A. J. Stunkard, Chairman of Psychiatry at the University of Pennsylvania.

If you want to change your eating habits to lose weight, he suggests that you keep a record of the amount of food you eat as well as the time and place. Limit your eating geography. Eat only in the kitchen or dining room. Nowhere else. Make an effort to take smaller bites. Chew each bite thoroughly before swallowing. Reward yourself by buying a new item of clothing for every inch you remove from your waist!

If that sounds extravagant, compare it to the cost of illness coming from body abuse!

Exercise and Diet

Exercise should always accompany any attempt to lose weight by dieting. If it does not, as the excess fat melts away, the stretched body covering is left to hang in folds. The only way to avoid such loose, sagging skin is to practice body movements to tighten the skin and render it more pliable as it returns to a normal, less stretched condition. An overall exercise plan is advisable here.

In conjunction with exercise, which should be practiced *every day* to firm flabby skin, there is a lotion you can make and massage into the skin to help it regain tone and strength. But remember, it is exercise that really tones, and the massaging action does more than the lotion to improve tone.

Toning Lotion

Mix three tablespoons of rose water, orange flower water, or elderflower water with one teaspoon of tincture of benzoin and one tablespoon of fresh cucumber juice. Strain through gauze into a bottle and apply before retiring for the night, and each morning upon arising.

Rose water and orange flower water can be purchased in a gourmet shop. You can prepare elderflower water from blossoms obtained from a botanical supply house, herbalist's shop or health food store. The benzoin is sticky, so work carefully with it.

How to Diet

Many hefty people are unsuccessful in their attempts to lose weight simply because they don't know how to diet! Jean Mayer, Professor of Nutrition at Harvard, believes that people try but fail to lose weight because they do not observe the following rules:

(1) Count every calorie. Everything that goes into your mouth but water. (2) Know your calorie needs; based on sex, age and body size, plus whether you are active or sedentary in your life style. (3) Portions are important. Watch them. (4) The calories you drink count, too. Many people overlook liquid calories, assuming they don't count. (5) Use sources other than protein for your quota of calories, for some protein foods contain fat, at 270 calories per ounce of fat! (6) Decrease sugar and salt consumption. Sugar, as we know, offers empty calories without nutrients. Salt reduction will cut down on water retention in the tissues. (7) Use a variety of foods in order to obtain all essential nutrients and make every calorie count. (8) Use only lean foods. (9) Exercising uses up calories. (10) Weigh yourself every morning.

It is always wise to check with your doctor before embarking on a serious weight loss program. And don't be concerned with a daily weight loss. Check yourself on the scale each day, yes, but don't expect results every time you check. Just hang in there and you will lose weight, if you adhere to a sensible diet.

Some people attempt to lose weight by eating only one meal a day, and snacking for the other two meals. Snacking will certainly do you in (or out), so why try to limit yourself to one meal a day? If you are like the average dieter, you consume far more at this meal than is wise, and more than make up for the two skipped meals.

Calculate the number of calories you require and spread them out over a full day, with some form of exercise in between in order to work them off.

And snacking adds calories, too! A stable weight pattern can be held more easily, this way, than through an extreme approach that allows indiscriminate snacking.

Overweight Children

The overweight child is a source of great concern to parents who are not themselves overweight. They often find it difficult to put their child on a diet plan, since they have no need of such a regimen for themselves. The whole family must be treated as a unit, and any obese family members must not be regarded as separate entities, according to Dr. Jerome L. Knittle of Mt. Sinai School of Medicine, New York (*Internal Medicine News,* June 15, 1974). If food is a primary concern in a family and meals consist of large portions, then naturally a child is going to protest being isolated from this family interest.

The tendency to accumulate fat cells can be determined at the age of two, Dr. Knittle says. And once this pattern is detected in obese children, there appears to be no change. For treatment to be of value to the obese child as he matures, he must be treated before the increased number of fat cells is established. Never resort to a crash diet for a child, for it can impede his or her normal growth.

Overweight Teenagers

The chubby teenager often comes from an environment in which eating is an important activity. The mother of this family loves to cook, and tells her overweight daughter not to worry about diet, that she is a "growing girl" who needs to eat a lot. For the overweight teenager who can't say no to Mama's good cooking, cutting down on food portions is essential.

If you're too heavy, you are obviously taking in too much food right now, so your object is to consume less, and get at it right away. A mother is not helping her child when she encourages unnecessary food consumption. The ability to resist such urgings to consume more food than one requires is what separates the girls from the women.

In addition to cutting out all the extravagant calories, the overweight teenager should begin a course of daily exercises so that the overstretched stomach can get back into shape.

Overweight Mothers

Cooking for an appreciative family has its rewards. You are looked upon as a warm and loving mother. Perhaps no one mentions that you are also plump.

But you can enjoy the same gratitude and love without endangering your health and that of your family. It would be a challenge to any good cook to replace fattening foods with delicious, wholesome dishes. You might want to get Jane Kinderlehrer's *Confessions of a Sneaky Organic Cook* (Rodale Press). This clever woman managed to keep her family happy, and even healthy, by serving tasty nutritious foods they would have rebelled against on their own.

Many people have found it helpful to adopt an interesting hobby to replace the compulsive habit of reaching for food. Weight reducers are advised to find a handicraft that interests them and to work at it daily. L. Melvin Elting, D.O., suggests woodworking, macrame, mosaics, stained glass, or metal working (*Obesity/Bariatric Medicine,* No. 4, 1974). You could also try weaving, sewing, knitting—anything that keeps your hands busy. Dr. Elting finds these crafts stimulate an appetite to create with the hands and lessens the one to self-destruct.

Weight Gain in Later Life

The person who has been slender all her life may find to her dismay that she begins to gain weight when she reaches the middle years, even though she has not increased her food intake. Seems terribly unfair, doesn't it? Just when you think you are free of dieting problems, up rears the ugly head of sedentary living. As one ages, the body requires fewer calories, and if you persist in consuming the same meal portions, you will find the bathroom scales tipping out of your favor. It is estimated that the body requires 16 percent fewer calories between the ages of 55 and 75 than previously.

Consider daily exercise and more moderate food consumption as the formula to remain lean and healthy at 55 and later.

One of the most beautiful women I've ever seen has remained slender and erect into her sixties. Genevieve had lived most of her life in North Africa, and developed a weight problem there. When she was widowed, she returned to her native Paris and found herself out of step with the slender Parisiennes. She tailored her diet to her actual needs and began walking morning and evening through the Bois de Boulognes, those beautiful woods called "the largest green space of Paris."

All that walking, plus giving up the delicious *couscous,* a fattening North African dish made from wheat, meat and beans, turned Genevieve into a stunning woman, more attractive than she had ever been in her life.

I visited Genevieve last year in Paris, and she prepared a dinner that was memorable, and which helped explain the perfectly shaped body of which she is justifiably proud. The lemon-roasted chicken had a sprinkling of toasted sesame seeds. The famous *haricots verts,* or green beans, so slender and tasty, were combined with minced basil and onion. A salad of spinach leaves and tomatoes followed, and a dessert of fresh fruit completed the meal.

Genevieve has had several proposals of marriage since she returned to her native city. And not because she is rich. In fact, Genevieve considers her lack of wealth a contributing factor to being slim. When funds are lean, one learns to dine on *morceaux,* or bits, rather than hefty chunks.

Creeping Obesity

The sinister shadow of creeping obesity sneaks up on more and more Americans each day. Creeping obesity is the tendency to gain weight because of poor dietary habits, rather than from an inheritance of a larger number of fat cells. Restrictive diets and vigorous exercise will bring about weight loss if adhered to. But if you abandon your diet and exercise after you've reached your goal, your size will gradually increase again. For weight loss to be fully effective, all dietary practices contributing to weight gain must be eliminated.

Yogurt

Yogurt is perhaps the most popular of all "diet" foods. Most types of yogurt are fairly low in calories, but it is wrong to assume that all kinds contain the same amount of calories. Yogurts vary in calorie count anywhere from 130 calories per cup for plain yogurt, to close to 300 calories for those sweetened with jams and preserves.

In addition to the added calories in the flavored varieties, the amount of sugar contained in the jams used to sweeten yogurt is a disadvantage. Try making your own yogurt from skim milk or buy it plain and add fresh fruit to it. Chopped apples, raisins or bananas are delicious combined with yogurt.

Fibrous Foods and Weight Loss

In the proper amounts, food fibers are supposed to prevent obesity. According to this theory, even if your food intake is comparatively small, if you are eating refined foods with the fibers processed out (white flour, for example, has the bran removed) you can easily gain weight (*Lancet,* January 19, 1974).

The value of food fibers in the diet would lie in (1) enhancing available nutrients in the diet, (2) fibers require lots of chewing, which promotes secretion of saliva and gastric juices which distend the stomach and promote satiety. Hence, you will feel full sooner and eat less. (3) Fiber reduces the absorptive efficiency of the small intestine; your body absorbs only what it needs, and eliminates the rest.

Group Therapy

There can be no blanket statement about the many clubs, farms and spas that promote weight loss. I am sure they do not "cure" every obese person who joins them, but many people have been helped by this type of group approach.

Self-help classes have proved their worth in many instances. Compulsive overeating is a disease which affects the person on three levels; physical, spiritual, and emotional (*Obesity/Bariatric Medicine,* No. 4, 1974). Willpower can be strengthened in a group approach to help surmount the emotional hurdle. A spirit of cooperation and involvement seems to be the persuasive element, plus the positive and approving attitudes of the group when weight loss is achieved.

Questions have been raised by medical people over the injections given in some of the anti-obesity clinics to aid in weight reduction. HCG, human chorionic gonadotropin, a growth hormone secreted in the urine of pregnant women, has been hailed by its devotees as a great help in attacking accumulations of abnormal fat in different body areas. Dr. Wilmer L. Asher, executive director of the American Society of Bariatric Physicians, says his group, along with other medical people including the AMA, are violently opposed to the use of HCG in weight reducing clinics.

There are differing reports from doctors who have given the HCG injections to their own patients. Some say that the restricted diet accompanying the injections is the important factor. Others say there is a striking redistribution of weight with its use. Many feel the hormone is useful simply as a placebo (*Medical World News,* October 11, 1974).

Hypnosis

Hypnosis has been used to help people lose weight. If you are receptive to controlled thought it can help you curb your desire for food. But what it cannot do is make you retain the new weight loss, for it does not cure the cause of overweight.

If your overeating stems from a compulsive action, you may simply substitute another self destructive behavior like smoking, or drinking, when you give up the compulsive eating. There are safer ways.

Acupuncture

People who have difficulty shedding extra pounds are ever on the prowl for a new way out of their weight problem. And who can blame them? However, care should be taken to avoid damaging the body with extreme dieting approaches. Occasionally an interesting, though bizarre, method is proposed for the unsuccessful dieter.

One such novel idea is to insert a staple-like needle in each ear. According to Dr. Frank Warren, hundreds of doctors are now employing this unique treatment for overweight. The staple-like insertions are placed in the ears because of nerve endings there which link various body areas to the brain. Their placement supposedly depresses the nerve which relates to the patient's desire for food.

Claiming a 70 percent rate of success in the 100 patients he has treated, Dr. Ellyn, an anesthesiologist in Encino, California, says this method is painless, and leaves no side effects. Dr. Warren states that when compulsive behavior is responsible for overeating it is usually a symptom of an underlying psychological disorder, which should receive separate treatment. Otherwise a patient cured of food craving may switch to other unhealthy habits like heavy smoking or alcoholism.

Jogging to Lose Weight

Exercise should always accompany a weight loss program unless otherwise decided by a doctor. But an overweight person newly embarked on a diet to lose weight should use a moderate approach to exercise, and avoid the strenuous exertion involved in an activity like jogging.

If she has been driving, she should begin walking more and using stairs instead of elevators. These suggestions were presented by Dr. Henry A. Jordan at a symposium sponsored by the Institute of Human Nutrition and the College of Physicians and Surgeons, at Columbia University in New York (*Family Practice News,* February 15, 1974).

Yoga exercises are excellent for tightening slack flesh. So are swimming and bicycling. Put off the jogging until you have reached your ideal weight.

Underweight

Although it may be hard to accept in the face of our modern tendency to associate beauty with extreme slenderness, underweight is as serious a problem as overweight. If you are unable to gain weight, first check with your doctor to be sure your condition has no medical origin. Instead of increasing the amount of food consumed at each meal, try increasing the number of meals you eat, to include five or six meals a day; this has helped many underweight people. Lie down and treat yourself to a blender drink made of milk, molasses, whole egg and banana. Whenever possible, rest for periods of time 'during a meal, by lying down before returning to the table.

Choose your food carefully, eliminating junk food, but concentrating on milk, eggs, cheese, meats and poultry, and also fresh fruits and vegetables.

In addition, you may require more exercise! After a 15 week exercise program conducted at the Preventive Medicine Center in Palo Alto, California, Jack H. Wilmore, Ph.D., Director of Physiological Evaluation at the Center, reported to the *Medical Tribune* in May, 1972, that seven women classified as chronically underweight showed an increase in body weight and lean body weight, with a decrease in absolute and relative fat.

Dr. Wilmore says meaningful weight gains can occur in chronically underweight women as a result of increased physical activity, just as it aids those who are overweight. The reason for success is the possible relationship of both conditions to an endocrine-metabolic balance.

Chapter 11

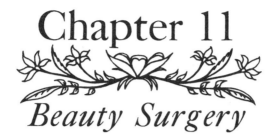

Beauty Surgery

Today, many women are adding cosmetic surgery to their lists of body upkeep practices. Once the domain of actors and actresses, this type of reconstructed beauty is becoming more accessible to women grown discontented with sagging jowls, overhanging lids, and drooping cheeks.

Preventive body care might have kept you from a premature need of cosmetic surgery. But if you were too busy to save a bit of time for daily body care, then a well recommended and highly capable cosmetic surgeon may be the answer to those crevasses and wattles. This type of all-out rebuilding does serve a need in today's youth-oriented world, in which the obviously aging are cast aside in favor of the young.

To those who might protest that this is not the "natural" approach to living which I am known to advocate, I say that if cosmetic surgery permits you to function more fully as a person, then there should be no question about its usefulness. We must never overlook the importance of good mental health and a comfortable attitude to every individual.

If one is born with defective or unattractive features which cause psychological pain, then whatever safe methods are available to alleviate these conditions should be considered therapeutic. I believe in a sensible, eyes-open attitude toward life, and would never back away from something that makes a person more secure and appreciative of herself, as long as no physical or psychological harm is involved.

If a person finds herself aging physically at too fast a clip for her purposes in life, and if this is depressing enough to destroy her pleasure in living, then cosmetic surgery should be able to help her.

When to Have Cosmetic Surgery

Most plastic surgeons shy away from women who restlessly look for "something new." After all, plastic surgery is *not* like going to the hairdresser, so it should not be considered casually.

The value of a change in facial structure lies in improvement of a disfiguring or unattractive feature, not in its chances of changing your life. Bernard E. Simon, M.D., Clinical Professor of Surgery at Mt. Sinai School of Medicine in New York and Chief of the Division of Plastic Surgery there, reported to *Hospital Practice* in July, 1972 that questions should be asked before accepting a patient for cosmetic surgery. For example, is the "defect" discernible to others than the patient? Is the patient seeking a solution to personal problems that really do not relate to facial appearance?

If you are considering plastic surgery simply because you want a new look, and not because of any real defect, reassess your problems and desires. This does not mean that cosmetic surgery should be limited only to a certain group. If it will improve your feeling of comfort with yourself and you are aware of all matters pertaining to the undertaking, and if your surgeon feels you are a good risk and your request is reasonable, then cosmetic surgery can be beneficial.

The middle aged woman who is exhibiting increasing signs of age may suddenly wish to have cosmetic surgery to make up for the years when she didn't take the time to care for her appearance. The woman who finds herself in this situation must carefully consider her motives for desiring surgery. What is her life style? Why is she concerned to the point of contemplating plastic surgery now, when for the years behind her, she was not concerned enough about her appearance to use the conventional methods to keep her body in good shape? Will a good diet plan and personal rehabilitation give her sufficient results to bring satisfaction? Is she in the business or professional world where keeping a youthful appearance is sometimes job insurance?

My point is that you must approach cosmetic surgery from an intelligent, sensible appraisal of your needs and desires, rather than as a whim to be "made over." Plastic surgery can solve many problems, but it will not guarantee you a better life, more security or endless youth.

If your mental attitude is stable, and you want to appear more attractive, then cosmetic surgery should prove beneficial. But you must realize that even after successful surgery, if you don't find time to take care of yourself, results can be disappointingly brief.

The Face

Dermabrasion, the removal of the scar tissue left by severe cases of acne, is a very useful procedure, as it removes between 50 and 70 percent of the scars on the area treated. It is considered safe when performed by an accredited physician, and the appearance of the skin is indeed greatly improved. The process is simple, only a bit uncomfortable, and endorsed as a medical procedure. A dental brush or burr abrades the skin surface, lessening, as it does, the pit depth of the pores and cutting down the raised scar tissue. A period of time is required afterwards for healing the newly exposed skin, and unguents are applied to help the process. It is considered quite beneficial for those afflicted with facial scar tissue.

The Eyes

The blepharoplasty is a special surgical procedure to correct baggy eyelids. This two to three hour operation can indeed do wonders for those suffering sagging lid tissue, baggy undereye areas, and to a degree, it can even remove crow's feet. The excess skin is surgically removed and the area resewn. Because a surgeon follows the natural crease of the eyelid, this form of cosmetic surgery is undiscernible after healing.

My neighbor had a blepharoplasty five years ago, and no sagging has recurred. However, this is still an area of delicate surgery, for two hazards are involved with the operation. Improper surgery can prevent the upper lid from closing, or the eyelid may droop permanently without being able to be raised. If this occurs, skin grafts are required for correction.

The Ears

The child with large, prominent ears is often the object of taunts and ridicule by his young classmates. As a result, many parents wish to have their children's ears surgically altered to spare the youngsters social embarrassment. This aspect of cosmetic surgery is generally acknowledged to be beneficial, but carries with it a greater possibility of infection or blood clotting than with the facial area. Called otoplasty, minimizing the size or shape of the ears requires reshaping of the cartilage of which the ear is composed. Performed by a competent surgeon, the dangers are minimized. The doctor will decide at what age to perform such a corrective procedure, but it is my understanding it can be performed very early in life.

This is an operation that reflects current trends, too. When fashion dictates that coiffures are swept back, or up, Dr. Nicholas G. Georgiade of Duke University Medical Center in North Carolina says he gets an influx of female patients asking to have their ears pinned back.

The Nose

Among the most common types of cosmetic surgery is the rhinoplasty, or "nose bob," as it is commonly known. This operation is considerably less dangerous than some other forms of surgery, which probably is one reason for its popularity. Infection is infrequent in rhinoplasty, and complications are relatively unknown.

Recovery is fairly rapid—after about three days in the hospital, a period of two weeks for general recovery follows. However, the nose may remain a bit swollen for a few months.

Rhinoplasty is performed on people of varying ages, but the surgeon will always be the one to decide whether the operation is advisable in a particular case. The surgery is not performed until after a person has reached his or her maximum growth (around 16 or 17). Costs vary according to the part of the country you are in, but generally the price ranges from $750 to $1,500 and up.

Some people are kept from having a rhinoplasty by the fear of damaging their new nose. And many others who do undergo the operation are driven by the same fear to give up sports and other activities they formerly enjoyed.

Physicians maintain that the belief that the nose is more fragile after surgery and subsequent full healing than before is completely unfounded. They point out the fact that a healed bone is equally as strong as a bone that has never been fractured. One can conclude, then, that any force strong enough to damage a healed bone would be equally likely to damage a normal bone.

The Breasts

Breast augmentation, one of the more controversial types of cosmetic surgery, is performed by plastic surgeons in most of the large cities in this country and abroad.

As with any form of surgery, one should not enter this procedure lightly. There should be a reasonable motivating factor. Several complications can arise from plastic surgery, including blood clots, excessive scarring, necrosis or sloughing off of the skin, and infection, but these after-effects may occur with any form of surgery.

Translucent silicone insertions are used by some surgeons to increase breast size. The surgeon slits the skin below each breast and places the artificial package behind the mammary gland.

Dr. Robert Alan Franklyn, a plastic surgeon in Hollywood, states that the breast itself is not operated on. Rather, breastplasty is a surgical procedure that is the equivalent of adding mass to the pectoral muscle in the back of the breast. So the mammary glands are not disturbed. Fear of cancer arising from breast implants meets an answer of "No" from medical men. Dr. Tibor de Cholnoky, Director of the Department of Plastic and Reconstructive Surgery at Greenwich Hospital in Connecticut, conducted a worldwide survey of mammary augmentations involving 10,941 cases as performed by 965 qualified plastic surgeons. After 18 years of follow-up study, no increase in cancer was reported among the patients involved.

Because the American Medical Association has issued a warning against the use of liquid silicone to inflate the breasts (it has caused several deaths), solid silicone, which does not migrate in the body as did the liquid, is being used instead.

Lower Body

The most common cause of excess flesh in the areas of the abdomen and thighs is overeating coupled with sedentary living habits. In most cases, diet and exercise provide the answer to this problem. However, some people find that no matter how much they curb their food intake, and how many kinds of exercise they try, they are unable to get rid of the fatty deposits.

If you are one of these unlucky sufferers, a visit to the doctor is of the utmost necessity. He can diagnose your condition to ascertain whether or not you can help yourself to lose weight. If the problem is beyond your control, there is the possibility of a controversial cosmetic operation that many medical men do not look upon strictly as a cosmetic improvement.

Performed infrequently in this country because of the extensive scarring, when surgery is warranted as the only means of removing grotesque amounts of body fat in the abdomen and thigh areas, surgeons do perform the lipodystrophia operation.

Dr. Thomas J. Baker, Jr., a Miami plastic surgeon,

describes the procedure he uses in *Medical World News,* September 11, 1970. While the patient is under general anesthesia he makes a crescent-shaped incision following the arc of the thigh crease, running from hip bone to hip bone. He then proceeds to pull up the apron of tissue and scoop out excess skin, fat and subcutaneous tissue. Dr. Baker then smooths out the trimmed area and closes the incision.

A similar procedure employing the same technique is used to alter the line of the buttocks. This is called a body lift, and like lipodystrophia, is not often performed in the United States because of the heavy scarring. Scarring is especially a drawback in the case of the buttocks because the operation leaves a seven- to eight-inch scar in a sensitive area which gets a lot of friction. The scarring can prove to be quite uncomfortable, and this type of operation should never be considered as a means of simply reducing excess weight.

Chapter 12

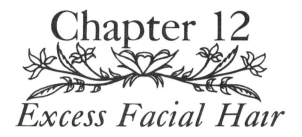

Excess Facial Hair

Some cases of excess body and facial hair indicate a disorder of the pituitary or adrenal glands, and medical aid should be sought. There is help at hand, if you will search until you find a doctor who realizes that your problem is not one of vanity.

A typical tragedy of yesterday would be avoidable today. According to Harriet Hubbard Ayer, a nineteenth century beauty advisor, a young girl of her acquaintance went into a decline and died because her puritanical father said if she had whiskers on her chin and face, it was because the Lord had intended it, and she must accept it.

The growth of excess facial hair seems to coincide with the menopausal period. However, a girl of 20 can also develop this unhappy condition, the same as a woman of 50. Some gynecologists say it is coincidental that hair growth appears at the same time oral hormones are being taken. They say that excess hair growth can be hereditary, and point to some women of European and Mediterranean descent as being more prone to this condition. It is the belief of gynecologists I have consulted that female hormones, taken to combat discomforts of the menopause, do not cause excess facial hair growth, though they all say there can be exceptions to the rule.

On the other hand, Dr. Howard McQuarrie of Western Gynecological and Obstetrical Clinic in Salt Lake City, Utah, suggests that a woman using oral contraceptives who suffers from abnormal hairiness (hypertrichosis), or who develops the condition while taking the Pill, should request a highly estrogenic type of oral contraceptive, and avoid the estrogen-free or progesterone dominant types (*Family Circle,* January, 1975).

A bugaboo to those affected, superfluous hair growth can generally be coped with by electrolysis, or less permanently, by other methods, when it is confined to the chin and upper lip area. However, all methods of removal other than electrolysis are of a temporary nature.

The electrolysis method, for safety's sake, requires a trained operator to perform the work. The operator inserts a fine needle driven by electric current into the hair follicle and attempts to destroy the hair root.

The electric needle should permanently destroy each root it touches, but sometimes there is regrowth. Return trips are required to treat these areas. Hair removal by electrolysis cannot be completed in a single visit to an operator. According to the amount of hair to be removed, several sessions over a period of weeks or months may be required to do a thorough job.

The do-it-yourself electrolysis approach seems unwise to me, and can result in pitted skin. A deft, delicate and knowledgeable touch is required for this, and you would be well advised to seek professional help rather than to go jabbing a piece of equipment into your skin hoping you will hit the right spot.

Choose your operator carefully. I've seen both good and bad results among friends who had hair removed by electrolysis. One attractive woman in New York had to have dermabrasion on her chin after electrolysis by an unskilled operator caused deep pit marks. Another friend in Washington, D.C. enjoyed terrific results. The New York friend saw an advertisement and visited the electrolysis operator, who apparently had bought the piece of equipment and set herself up in business without prior training. The woman in Washington chose her operator on the recommendation of a friend. It is my belief that a well known department store would engage only highly skilled operators and one would be quite safe there, though there are, of course, reliable independent operators as well.

To remove or disguise excess hair on the arms and legs, less permanent methods are often used. Wax depilatories are popular, but some women find this a painful and unsatisfactory method of hair removal. Depilatories do not destroy the root, but merely clear the area until new growth emerges.

Tweezing to remove excess hair can be done to isolated hairs on the facial surface. Obviously, it is not practical for arm, leg and underarm areas. Chemical depilatories which dissolve hair can be effective. But by their very nature of destroying the protein structure of the hair, these chemical compounds should be used with great caution since skin, also, is composed of protein and irritation or hardened surface skin could result.

Bleaches can be used, but remember that anything strong enough to strip away color from hair is also strong enough to irritate the skin. If you use this method of lightening hair on your arms or legs, be sure to wash the skin carefully afterwards and to use an acid rinse to restore the native acid mantle to the skin. Apple cider vinegar and water in an eight to one proportion (in favor of the water) is a good mixture.

Chapter 13

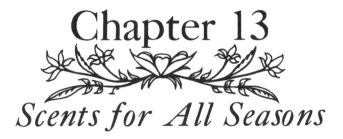

Scents for All Seasons

A book on beauty, to me, is not complete until it touches the soul, or inspires that part of the mind which interprets the messages of the senses. All our senses enable us to live more fully, experience more deeply, and learn more comprehensively.

Our early ancestors depended on their highly refined sense of smell to detect the presence of predatory animals and to find edible foods. However, in the process of evolution man's eyesight seemingly surpassed his sense of smell, and today we are so busy looking we greatly underestimate the importance of our olfactory sensations. Anyone who has lost her sense of smell during a bad cold can tell you what a dismal affair dining can become.

Montaigne, the French essayist, believed that the medical world could promote the cause of health by greater use of scents. Odors, he said, contain qualities to change one's attitudes and spirits, and according to the scent, can dramatically alter a person's mood.

We all know that beauty of the soul is mirrored on the body. It follows, then, that pleasing the soul by stimulating the senses can charm the physical body, too. Pleasing scents should have a secure place in everyone's life. Per-

haps the wonder of smell is the dimension of subtle pleasure it opens to us, and therefore it could be called a luxury
sense, though practical in its services. By refining this
acuity, you can greatly increase the beauty and felicity of
your days.

In your own home you can experiment and put together
enchanting fragrances that excite, stimulate, soothe, calm,
or put you into a soft, dreamy mood. This creative effort
can be immensely rewarding, for in moments of the greatest despondency, turning to the vital forces of nature never
fails to bring a sense of renewal.

The lavender you grow in your garden can be the basis
for your first project. This favored scent supposedly attracts the male. The women of ancient Rome who had a
reputation for being amorous used lavender oil in their
baths. But you need have in mind nothing more than an
appreciation for its lasting fragrance and its lulling, clean
scent to enjoy it.

Try the following mixture for a whiff of gentler times,
and more subtle scents, before the press of an aerosol button
could saturate the air with a chemical version of perfume.

LAVENDER SACHET

8 ounces	lavender flowers
8 ounces	orris root
4 ounces	benzoin gum
4 ounces	tonka beans
2 ounces	cloves
2 ounces	sandalwood
2 ounces	cinnamon
1 ounce	vanilla bean

Grind all the above ingredients to a powder and mix

well. Place in small drawstring bags. Tuck the sachets into drawers containing your clothing.

Small amounts of essential oils may be added to various combinations of solid perfume bearing materials (like flowers, herbs and stick spices) which are reduced to a powder before adding the oils.

Spicy Sachet

Another delicately scented sachet calls for one ounce each of the following items: cinnamon, cloves, coriander seeds, lavender flowers, rose leaves and orris root. All the ingredients are pulverized and ladled into small bags and tied.

Heliotrope is an old fashioned sachet powder, treasured as a lovely scent for bed linens and towels. It lends a nostalgic and delightful touch of the past to a modern day linen closet whose contents never get outside a laundry room. Modern day washers and driers are a great convenience, but don't supply the freshness of the sunsweet breeze that was a natural perfume of bed linens in the past.

Heliotrope Sachet

Grind one-half pound of orris root and add one-fourth pound ground rose petals, two ounces powdered tonka beans, one ounce vanilla bean, one-half teaspoon labdanum, and two drops of almond oil. Mix together by sifting through a coarse sieve, place in bags, and tuck among your sheets and towels.

I have replaced the musk fixative in the original formula with labdanum because a musk deer must be destroyed in order to obtain musk of animal origin. This Tibetan species is in danger of extinction because of the increased demand for the oil from glands of the male deer to be used in scent preparation. Labdanum is an excellent substitute and comes from a variety of rockrose shrubs.

Patchouli powder is one of the simpler, but very potent, scenting mixtures. This East Indian plant is native to the Malay peninsula, and has long been used in perfumery and cosmetics. The leaves and oil of the exotic plant are also effective as a deodorant. The haunting scent is considered one of the most provocative of all growing things, and can add a sense of mystery to your preparations.

Patchouli Sachet

Blend together one-fourth pound of ground patchouli and one-fourth pound of ground sandalwood. Add a few drops of patchouli oil and mix well before placing in suitable containers.

Fragrances can be caught in perfumes, sachets, oils, toilet water and colognes, but probably the most durable of all perfumery is found in the rose bowl. Petals can be dried and added to other lingering, spicy scents to provide pleasure for a dozen or more years. I've come across tightly covered old rose jars in antique shops that retained their delicate perfume for a quarter of a century.

In earlier times this collection of rose petals was called a sweet jar, and I have seen exquisite containers in the Baccarat Glass and Porcelain Museum on *rue Paradis* in Paris that were made especially for this purpose more than 200 years ago. But you can use a variety of pretty covered containers for your rose bowl. I prefer an old fashioned soup tureen and have a rose bowl that I started over five years ago. Every few weeks I remove the lid and the exquisite perfume of rose petals and oils fills the room.

Rose Bowl

During rose season on sunny days collect petals of any and all varieties of roses. Gather them as soon as the sun has dried the dew on the leaves. Strip the petals from the calyx, disposing of any decayed or blemished petals. When one gallon has been collected, take a porcelain bowl and alternate layers of petals and sea salt, so that the last layer is salt. Press down with a plate that can be left in the bowl. Turn the mixture after 12 hours. Very carefully stir the petals every day for a week. After the mass becomes moistened, add three ounces of ground allspice. For the next three days mix the petals and spice, and on each of those days add a quarter of an ounce each of allspice and ground cinnamon.

Now put the mixture into the jar, bowl, or other container you have chosen and add the following ingredients, all coarsely powdered: cloves, cinnamon, nutmeg, mace, allspice, orange and lemon peel, anise seed and root (one ounce each); black pepper, one-quarter ounce; one-half teaspoon labdanum. Finally, add one-half teaspoon rose geranium oil. Or use lavender or rosemary oil if you prefer.

Throughout the summer you may add any of your favorite petals, but dry them in the open air before adding. From time to time stir the mixture and leave the lid off so the perfume can fill the air. But keep the jar tightly closed for a month after each opening, to allow the scents to gather potency again.

You can achieve similar results by first drying the rose petals thoroughly and proceeding with the same ingredients listed for the moist method, with the same timing schedule for adding the spices and oils. To dry the rose petals, place them outdoors each day in the shade and bring them in each night. Keep them in a large basket and stir each day until they are fully dried before placing them in the rose bowl.

If you want to feel very special and if you've a yen for scents that are fresh and natural, put together your own scented waters. These are lightly fragrant waters, so expect a delicate waft of perfume. In earlier days heavy scents weren't considered in good taste, and this wasn't a bad idea. There is nothing quite so cloying and unpleasant as being in a crowded room where your senses are assaulted from all sides with many and varied heady perfumes. Everyone loses her perfume identity this way. But a light summer breeze of a scent that happens along in a group of packed bodies is a welcomed treat.

OLD COLONY SCENTED WATER

1 teaspoon	oil of lemon
1 teaspoon	oil of balm
1 teaspoon	oil of orange
2 teaspoons	oil of lavender
1½ teaspoons	oil of rosemary
10 drops	oil of rose
1 pint	ethyl alcohol

Mix all ingredients together in a glass jar and shake vigorously three times a day for a week, then strain through wet filter paper into smaller bottles.

Perfume

When applying perfume to the body, don't use it on areas where the sun can get to it. This can cause discoloration of the skin; when the sun's rays reach a perfumed skin area, the skin becomes highly sensitive, and you may be left with unattractive spotting and blotching. Use perfume, according to most manufacturers, in the pulse spots on the body. But avoid exposed areas.

The selection of perfume is an art. Your own body chemistry will dictate the scents most suited to you. In a little shop next door to the news agency where I worked in Paris, a knowledgeable perfume chemist reigned supreme. Women came from all over the city to have Madame la Parfumeuse apply a dab of perfume to the wrist, wave it about to dry, and then wait until the body reacted to the scent, pleasantly or otherwise. Also taken into consideration was the client's physical appearance—a petite, delicate woman dared the chemist's ire if she requested a heavy scent.

I learned my own perfume scent there, and have never really tired of it, for it helps express the light, faintly floral world I find so agreeable. When I prepare my own scents from various perfumed oils, I try to remain within a range of scents most nearly resembling the faintly fragrant, rather than a less subtle scent.

Many times a bath oil will serve the same purpose as perfume, is less costly to use because it lasts longer, and is less likely to irritate the skin. You can find these oils at cosmetic counters, or you might choose to order an essential oil from a cosmetic company or botanical supply house. Use as a perfume by dabbing it on the same pulse areas where you apply perfume. But, as with any scented product, avoid areas the sun can reach.

Appendix

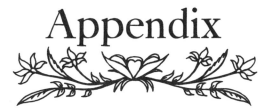

Stocking Your Beauty Cupboard

How to Care
For Your Body Every Day

Basic Beauty Foods
And
What They Do For You

What to Feed Your Body

Exercises For All Your Problem Areas

Where to Look For Supplies

Stocking Your Beauty Cupboard

Why not set aside a couple of shelves for your beauty supplies, and have them right at your fingertips whenever you need them!

These are the items you'll want to keep on hand:

Mineral water

Mineral water has no added chemicals or pollutants. In effect, it is "pure" water.

Natural vegetable, seed, or nut oils

The best oils to use are polyunsaturated and cold pressed. Try corn, safflower, olive, soy, sesame and apricot. The place most likely to stock cold pressed oils is a health food shop.

Honey

Raw, unfiltered honey comes in many varieties, both light and dark. It is somewhat cloudy in appearance, and of course, contains no sulfur. Shop for this type of honey at a roadside stand, a local farmers' market, a health food store or mail order suppliers.

Apple cider vinegar

Cider vinegar is preferable to white or wine vinegars (which are further distilled) for use in beauty preparations. It's easy to store, and is available in supermarkets.

Brewer's yeast

This is a special type of yeast in which the yeast organisms are no longer alive. Be sure to use only brewer's yeast, because the active yeast used in baking can be a threat to nutritional stores when eaten raw or externally applied. You'll find brewer's yeast in its versatile powder form in health food stores.

Almonds

Raw, unshelled almonds are available in most supermarkets and other grocery outlets. It's best to buy them unshelled to be sure of freshness. They can also be stored longer when the shells are left intact.

Powdered skim milk

No problem to store, convenient to use, and available in any food market—powdered skim milk is a must for the well-stocked beauty cupboard. The non-instant kind is preferable.

Oatmeal

Another universally available food; but please, don't buy the instant or quick-cooking kinds. You want to be sure you're getting all the vitamins and minerals contained in oatmeal, so use only the natural, unadulterated product. And good news—it's cheaper that way.

Mint

The mint family encompasses a wide variety of plants. Most common are peppermint and spearmint. Dried mint is available in most health food stores, but since it is so easy to do, why not grow your own to be assured of highest quality? Mint is a most delightful addition to a summer garden!

Rosemary

Chances are you already have rosemary in your kitchen. If you don't, make it a point to get a supply for cooking as well as for beauty needs. It's easy to grow your own rosemary, or you can purchase it at supermarkets, health food stores or herbal shops.

Sage

This pungent herb is one of the basics for your beauty cupboard. Like most of the other herbs on your shelf, you can grow sage in your garden, or purchase it dried in your local health food shop. If there are no natural food stores or herbal stores in your area, you might wish to purchase dried herbs from a mail order company (see "Where To Look for Supplies").

And in your refrigerator:
    whole milk
    eggs
    fresh lemons
    carrots
    tomatoes
    cucumbers

an assortment of fresh fruits and
vegetables suited to your own needs

These utensils will come in handy in concocting your
beauty preparations:

Mortar and pestle

Old fashioned, but still the best way to grind fresh or
dried foods to a pulp, meal or powder.

Small glass bottles

An assortment of tightly covered vials is indispensable
to the kitchen cosmetician. You'll need them to bottle
facial lotions, shampoos, bath mixtures, hand creams and
colognes. Save your glass medicine bottles, baby food jars,
spice containers—any small bottle that closes tightly. Start
your own personal recycling program.

Blender

For those who, for lack of time or energy, want the easy
way out, a blender is truly a luxury machine. It can whip,
chop or grind whatever you need in a matter of seconds.

Cheesecloth

This loosely woven fabric is excellent for straining
coarse matter from your lotions and potions. It is also the
best material to use for bath bags of herbs and flowers.

Cotton balls

Keep a good supply on hand for smoothing on facial

lotions, astringents and makeup removers, and for blotting excess oils and creams from your face and hands.

Gauze squares

These may be used to strain lotions, and for convenience in applying facials.

Wooden spoons

The best type of spoon to use in mixing and beating your homemade cosmetics. A wooden spoon is particularly helpful when you're working with hot preparations, since it will not conduct heat as does a metal spoon.

Measuring spoons

Some of the cosmetic recipes in this book call for exact amounts of ingredients, so measuring spoons are a must. You might like to buy an extra set; use one for making beauty foods and one for preparing external beauty care concoctions.

White washcloths

For any compress-type application, when you are required to keep a wet cloth over your face for a period of time, a white washcloth is the best thing to use. Many of these applications will stain the cloth, so you may want to reserve it only for compresses.

Natural bristle hairbrush

By far the best kind to use to keep your hair healthy and shining. Natural bristles won't scratch the scalp surface as nylon bristles do, and are gentler to your hair.

Complexion brush

This small brush is specially designed for cleansing delicate facial skin. The bristles deep clean the pores without pulling on the skin as does a washcloth.

Loofah mitt

The loofah mitt, or massage glove, is made from the fibers of a special type of gourd. When rubbed lightly over the body, the loofah mitt carries away dead cells and debris from the skin surface. The friction created by its rough texture stimulates the circulation to revive a weary body.

How to Care
For Your Body Every Day

Here are some suggestions for preparations you'll want to use regularly for your particular type of skin and hair. Experiment, choose your favorites, and keep them on hand to look your very best.

For Your Skin

Normal Skin

Cleansers: almond meal, oatmeal, oatmeal and cream
General care lotions: milk of roses, cucumber milk lotion, strawberries and cream, coconut oil, elderflower water
General care masks: fresh strawberry, strawberry and cream, cucumber, Fuller's Earth
Bath enrichers: oatmeal, bran, milk, rosemary, sage, mint, rose geranium, lavender, plantain leaves, blackberry leaves

Dry Skin

Cleansers: almond meal, milk, oatmeal, oatmeal and cream, bran, grape

Special care lotions: oil and lanolin, honey treatments
Special care masks: puree of carrot, corn, wheat germ,
    sesame oil
Bath enrichers: bran, oatmeal, milk, oil

Oily Skin

Cleansers: almond meal, cornmeal, lime juice
Special care lotions: lemon water, witch hazel or
    herbal astringents, skim milk makeup remover
Special care masks: brewer's yeast, pear or water-
    melon facial, Fuller's Earth
Bath enrichers: oatmeal, vinegar

Mosaic Skin

Cleansers: almond meal, oatmeal
Special care facials:
    oily areas—lemon/egg facial
    dry areas—gelatin facial
Bath enrichers: oatmeal, herbs

Blemished Skin

Cleansers: almond meal, cornmeal
Special care lotion: parsley
Special care masks: carrot, dock poultice
Facial steams: papaya, papaya-mint, burdock

Dull Skin

Cleansers: almond meal, cornmeal
Special care masks: pineapple, fresh or dried apricot,
    wheat germ, brewer's yeast

Friction scrubs: sunflower meal, cornmeal
Types of baths: salt, dry bath (with loofah mitt)

Mature Skin

Cleansers: almond meal, oatmeal, oatmeal and cream
Special care lotions: elderflower water, watercress lotion, benzoin firming lotion
Special care masks: brewer's yeast
Wrinkle-chasers: egg white and lemon juice, banana, oatmeal and cream

For Your Hair

Normal Hair

Shampoos: herbal, soapbark, castile

Dry Hair

Shampoos: lanolin, egg
Special care: avocado conditioner, protein conditioner, "Shimmer and Shine Hair Gloss"

Oily Hair

Shampoos: herbal, soapbark, castile
Special care: lime scalp cleanser

Damaged Hair

Shampoos: herbal, egg yolk
Special care conditioners: castor oil pack, mayonnaise, hydrolyzed protein, molasses, honey

Controlling Your Hair

Lemon hair spray; quince seed, flaxseed, rosemary or skim milk setting lotions

Tints

Blonde: camomile, egg white, lemon juice, ale

Brunette: henna/camomile, henna/sage, walnut, sage/black tea, tag alder bark

Basic Beauty Foods
And
What They Do For You

Food	External Properties
Almond	cleansing, smoothing, soften ing
Benzoin	stimulating, antiseptic
Blackberry Leaves	astringent
Bran	nourishing, softening

Food Value	*How To Use It*
protein to rebuild skin, hair and nails; vitamin B to metabolize other nutrients, promote growth of hair and nails, for healthy skin, eyes, nerves, digestion; calcium to clear blemished skin, calm troubled nerves, strengthen bones and teeth; vital minerals	facial lotion, cleansing grains; blackhead cleanser; dry shampoo; scrub for dry knees; bath enricher
	skin toning lotions; fixative for sachets and scents
	lotion for distressed skin; bath enricher
protein to rebuild skin, hair and nails; vitamin B to metabolize other	cleanser for face and hands; bath enricher

Food	External Properties
Brewer's Yeast	cleansing, nourishing, tightening; activates circulation
Burdock	cleansing, healing
Cocoa Butter	emollient, softening
Cornmeal	cleansing, friction-producin
Cucumber	cleansing, cooling, toning

Food Value	*How To Use It*
nutrients, promote growth of hair and nails; for healthy skin, eyes, nerves, digestion; calcium to clear blemished skin, calm troubled nerves, strengthen bones and teeth; vital minerals	
vitamin B to metabolize other nutrients, promote growth of hair and nails; for healthy skin, eyes, nerves, digestion; protein to rebuild skin, hair and nails	facial masks for oily, sallow or fatigued skin; wrinkle-chaser
	steam facial for blemished skin
	moisturizer for dry skin; stretch mark preventive
vitamin A for healthy skin, eyes, mucous membranes; vitamin B to metabolize other nutrients, promote growth of hair and nails; for healthy skin, eyes, nerves, digestion; vital minerals	scrub for dull skin; bath enricher
vitamin C for healthy connec-	lotion for oily complexion;

271

Food	External Properties
Dock	astringent, blood cooling
Egg	tightening, nourishing
Elderflower	soothing, bleaching
Fuller's Earth	toning, stimulating
Grapes	nourishing, cleansing
Honey	softening, nourishing, healir

Food Value	How To Use It
tive tissues, bones and cartilage; for repairing damaged cells; calcium to clear blemished skin, calm tense nerves, strengthen bones and teeth; vital trace minerals	toner for fatigued skin; undereye brightener, general care lotions and masks
	poultice for skin impurities and inflammations
vitamin A for healthy skin, and teeth; vitamin D for strong bones and teeth; protein to rebuild skin, hair and nails; iron to build red blood cells; vital minerals	skin toner; skin food; undereye tightener; wrinkle-chaser; shampoos for dandruff, dry or damaged hair; conditioners
	lotion for rough, sensitive or mature skin
	facial masks
vitamin A for healthy skin, eyes, mucous membranes; vital minerals	cleanser for dry or oily skin
natural bactericide to soothe irritations; vital minerals	lip balm; hair conditioner; for flaky legs and dry elbows

Food	External Properties
Lemon	astringent, acidic, refreshing, bleaching
Milk	nourishing, cleansing, softening
Mint	cleansing, refreshing, soothing
Oatmeal	cleansing, softening, nourishing

Food Value	*How To Use It*
vitamin C for healthy bones, cartilage and connective tissue; for repairing damaged cells; vitamin A for healthy skin, eyes, mucous membranes	facial lotion for oily skin; hair rinse; hair spray; hair lightener; tooth whitener; hand cleanser; restores skin's acid mantle
vitamin D for strong bones and teeth; calcium to clear blemished skin, calm tense nerves, strengthen bones and teeth; phosphorus to burn fats and starches; vital minerals	face cleanser; makeup remover; setting lotion; dry hand cream; bath enricher
	facial steam; summer skin refresher; bath enricher; internal cleanser
vitamin B to metabolize other nutrients, promote growth of hair and nails; for healthy skin, eyes, nerves, digestion; calcium to calm tense nerves, clear blemished skin, strengthen bones and teeth; iron to build red blood cells; vital minerals	face cleanser; wrinkle-chaser; bath enricher

Food	*External Properties*
Unsaturated Vegetable, Seed and Nut Oils	lubricating
Pineapple	enzymatic, rejuvenating
Plantain	astringent, soothing, heali
Rosemary	cleansing, stimulating, germ cidal, coloring
Sage	astringent, cleansing, invig rating, coloring
Strawberry	bleaching, softening, nouris ing
Tomato	bleaching, cleansing, stim lating

Food Value	*How To Use It*
unsaturated fats to lubricate and regenerate skin; aid circulation	facials for dry or suntanned skin; pre-bath rub for flaky skin; bath enricher
vitamin A for healthy skin, eyes, mucous membranes vitamin C for healthy bones, cartilage and connective tissues; for repairing damaged cells vital minerals	facials masks for dull complexion
	bath enricher
	hair rinse; bath enricher; internal cleanser
	astringent lotion; hair tint; bath enricher
vitamin A for healthy skin, eyes, mucous membranes; vitamin C for healthy bones, cartilage and connective tissue; for repairing damaged cells; vital minerals	facial lotions and masks
vitamin A for healthy skin, eyes, mucous membranes; vitamin C for healthy bones, cartilage, and connective tis-	facials for oily, dull or darkened skin

Food	*External Properties*
Wheat Germ	nourishing, softening
Witch Hazel	astringent, refreshing, germ cidal, stimulating
Yogurt	bleaching

Food Value	*How To Use It*
sue; for repairing damaged cells vital minerals	
protein to rebuild skin, hair and nails; vitamin B to metabolize other nutrients, promote growth of hair and nails; for healthy skin, eyes, nerves, digestion; vitamin E to preserve oxygen within body, improve cell function; helps other vitamins to be absorbed by body	facial mask for dry or dull skin; bath enricher
	astringent lotions
protein to rebuild skin, hair and nails; vitamin A for healthy skin, eyes, mucous membranes; helps intestinal tract to manufacture vitamin B; calcium to clear blemished skin, calm troubled nerves, strengthen bones and teeth; ·minerals	facials for oily, dull or discolored skin

What to Feed Your Body

"You are what you eat"—there is indeed a measure of truth to the old adage. Regular intake of different kinds of foods is reflected by your body in skin and hair conditions, and in weight gains or losses. While you are caring for your body's external needs, consider also how your diet can help to solve (or create) beauty problems.

The first requirement for health and beauty is a well balanced diet, containing all the vital nutrients in proportions tailored to your physical frame, age, sex and lifestyle. Very basically, aim for a diet that includes a variety of foods from the four major food groups—meats and fish, dairy products, fruits and vegetables, grain products. Feed your skin the same nutrients the rest of your body needs.

Generally speaking, foods that cause problems for healthy skin and hair are the same foods that may harm a healthy body. Try to avoid refined sugar, saturated animal fats, fried or heavily processed foods, and all kinds of junk foods.

Listed below are some foods that should be emphasized in a well balanced diet plan to help clear up specific problems.

The Skin

Oily Skin

Helpful foods—fresh fruits and vegetables (and their juices), fish, poultry, lean meats, eggs, whole grain cereals

Supplemental suggestions—brewer's yeast

Dry Skin

Helpful foods—polyunsaturated vegetable, seed or nut oils, protein-rich foods

Supplemental suggestions—vitamins A and E

Dull or Muddy Skin

Helpful foods—yogurt, apricots

Supplemental suggestions—brewer's yeast, vitamin B complex

Blemished Skin

Helpful foods—fresh green vegetables, almonds, sunflower seeds, wheat germ, cranberry juice, cucumbers, liver, carrots, sweet potatoes, apricots

Supplemental suggestions—vitamins A, B-complex, and E, bone meal or calcium lactate, lecithin, magnesium

The Hair

Oily Hair

Helpful foods—fresh fruits and vegetables, fish, poul-

try, lean meats, whole grain cereals
Supplemental suggestions—vitamin B-complex, vitamin A

Dry Hair

Helpful foods—one to two tablespoons unprocessed vegetable, seed or nut oil each day, cod-liver oil
Supplemental suggestions—vitamin E, vitamin A

Dandruff

Helpful foods—liver, cod-liver oil, unsaturated vegetable oils, wheat germ, fresh fruits and vegetables, protein-rich foods
Supplemental suggestions—desiccated liver, brewer's yeast, bone meal, lecithin

Fading Color

Helpful foods—liver, wheat germ, blackstrap molasses, sunflower seeds, whole grain cereals, rice polish, seafood, yogurt, cold-pressed vegetable and nut oils
Supplemental suggestions—brewer's yeast, kelp, vitamin B-complex

The Eyes

Helpful foods—leafy green and yellow vegetables, wheat germ, rice polish, molasses, sunflower seeds
Supplemental suggestions—vitamins A, B-complex,

C, D and E, brewer's yeast, bone meal or calcium lactate

The Teeth

Helpful foods—crusty and fibrous foods, raw, crisp vegetables, fresh fruits

Supplemental suggestions—vitamins A, C and D, bone meal

The Nails

Helpful foods—almonds, liver, blackstrap molasses, apricots, eggs, wheat germ, whole grain cereals, protein foods, horsetail tea

Supplemental suggestions—vitamin A, brewer's yeast. zinc, calcium lactate

The Overweight Torso

Helpful foods—fresh fruits, raw vegetables, sunflower seeds, apricots, dates, yogurt, fibrous foods

The Underweight Torso

Helpful foods—milk, eggs, cheese, meats, poultry, fresh fruits and vegetables

Exercises
for All Your Problem Areas

What It Helps	Exercise
Eyes (crow's feet)	wink 'n' smile
Eyes (fatigue)	glance-about
Eyes (fatigue)	focused head roll
Face	the lion
Underchin	the turtle
Neck	head rotations
Neck	head roll
Back	press to wall
Back	curl-up roll
Spine	puppet
Swayback	back alignment
Swayback	knee raise/arm fling
Swayback	back stretch
Upper Back	the cat
Bust	toner
Bust	hand press
Waist	circling
Abdomen	alternate leg raise
Abdomen	contractions

What It Does	Where To Find It
reduces lines	page 125
strengthens eye muscles	page 129
relaxes strained muscles	page 130
tones facial muscles	page 221
tones and tightens	page 167
loosens	page 167
relaxes stiffness	page 168
flexes back muscles	page 170
limbers stiff muscles	page 171
straightens the spine	page 172
straightens spine to properly distribute weight	page 173
strengthens back muscles	page 173
strengthens back muscles	page 173
tones and reduces	page 174
firms and tones	page 175
firms and tones	page 175
trims	page 176
firms and trims	page 177
firms and flattens	page 178

What It Helps	Exercise
Hips	knee bounce
Hips	side leg lift
Torso	body circles
Upper Arms	the bow
Upper Arms	lifting the box
Lower Body	knee pulls
Thighs	leg stretch
Thighs	kneel 'n' sit
Legs and Pelvis	squatting
Legs and Pelvis	kneel 'n' sit
Knees	toe curl
Knees	knee bends
Ankles	foot circles
Feet	rolling pin rolls
Feet	wall walking
Feet	rocking foot balance
Whole Body	the ball
Whole Body	complete breath
Whole Body	alternate breathing

What It Does	Where To Find It
limbers	page 222
trims	page 179
stretches and invigorates	page 220
firms and tones	page 180
firms and tones	page 180
stretches and invigorates	page 220
firms and trims	page 186
tones and trims	page 186
flexes and limbers	page 219
flexes and limbers	page 219
tones and strengthens	page 189
tones	page 190
trims	page 190
strengthens and relaxes	page 191
strengthens and relaxes	page 191
strengthens arch	page 191
relaxes	page 218
calms and relaxes	page 216
calms and relaxes	page 216

Where to Look for Supplies

Caswell-Massey Company, Ltd.
518 Lexington Avenue
New York, New York 10021
   This distinguished firm handles herbs, spices, perfumes and potpourris. For a catalogue, send one dollar to them at 320 West 13th Street, New York, New York 10014

Caprilands Herb Farm
Silver Street
Coventry, Connecticut 06238
   You can have many kinds of herbs from these gardens, and lovely sachets and potpourris.

Hausmann's Pharmacy
6th and Girard Avenue
Philadelphia, Pennsylvania 19123
   This old-time drugstore is filled with herbs, spices and essential oils.

Indiana Botanic Gardens
Hammond, Indiana 46325

An established supplier offering a variety of herbs, natural remedies, oils and gum resins.

Nature's Herb Company
281 Ellis Street
San Francisco, California 94102

All kinds of herbs, flowers and essential oils. You can request a price list from the company.

Index

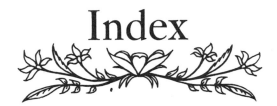

The Handbook of Natural Beauty